A SURGICAL REVOLUTION

A SURGICAL REVOLUTION

Surgery in Scotland, 1837–1901

PETER F. JONES

First published in Great Britain in 2007 by John Donald, an
imprint of Birlinn Ltd

West Newington House
10 Newington Road
Edinburgh
EH9 1QS

www.birlinn.co.uk

ISBN 10: 0 85976 684 5
ISBN 13: 978 0 85976 684 5

British Library Cataloguing-in-Publication data
A catalogue record for this book is available on request from the
British Library

Typeset by Carnegie Book Production, Lancaster
Printed and bound in Great Britain by Antony Rowe Ltd, Chippenham, Wiltshire

Contents

Introduction

During the sixty-four years of the reign of Queen Victoria (1837–1901), there were many outstanding industrial and scientific developments, among which must be counted the transformation of the practice of surgery.

Many have heard of Joseph Lister; they may use *Listerine*, and associate the name with the use of antiseptics. Relatively few know of his life, or the remarkable details of the discovery of the Antiseptic Principle. Even less is known of Lister's Scottish friends – Ogston, Macewen, Thomas Keith and James Simpson. Yet it is not too much to claim that their work was at the very forefront of 'a surgical revolution'.

In 1837 there was no general anaesthesia for the surgical patient. Only a few patients could bring themselves to face the pain of an operation and surgeons felt there had to be compelling reasons to inflict it. Moreover, there was no reliable way of preventing infection of the wound, which could frustrate the exercise of their skill. These hard old practices came to an end with the two great advances of the nineteenth century – general anaesthesia, and the conquest of surgical sepsis.

In 1846 ether was first used in New England to relieve the pain of dental and surgical operations, and in the following year Simpson in Edinburgh introduced the use of chloroform, which rapidly became a popular general anaesthetic. Surgery lost many of its terrors, but it was still not safe because so many surgical wounds, quite unpredictably, became septic, and this could lead to serious illness.

Then, twenty years later, in 1867, Joseph Lister was working in Glasgow, on ideas suggested by Pasteur, which would enable him to publish the results of two years of work which established the 'Antiseptic Principle in the Practice of Surgery'. When he moved to Edinburgh in 1869 Lister showed that observance of these principles allowed surgical operations to be performed cleanly and safely. They enabled William Macewen, Lister's student, to operate safely in the 1870s on some 300 Glasgow children who were crippled by bowed legs or knock-knees, restoring them to happy, healthy mobility.

At the same time, another friend of Lister's, Alex Ogston in Aberdeen, was pursuing the actual cause of surgical sepsis. Working in his laboratory, in a shed in the garden of his house in Union Street, he was able to isolate and identify the germ *Staphylococcus aureus*.

In the late nineteenth century abdominal surgery was generally considered to be unsafe, yet its potential was to be revealed by Thomas Keith, a general practitioner in Edinburgh. Working in the whitewashed attic of his house, he operated on 300 women to relieve them of the burden of carrying a large ovarian cyst: in the final group of 100 patients only three died.

It is important to study and appreciate the work of these pioneers in the light of the prevailing climate of opinion in which they lived. Each man had to place his trust in a new set of principles, and face a critical group of colleagues. Lister could only trust in his own recognition of the researches of Pasteur: when he dared to treat severe compound fractures conservatively with carbolic acid, rather than the customary amputation, he took a lonely, vulnerable path.

These were pioneering individuals, often working in unfavourable conditions, yet achieving remarkable results with simple instruments and apparatus of their own devising. The details of their lives which they left in their notes, letters and papers and in the recollections of their friends, present many memorable stories. In this account it is hoped that they will come to life in a straightforward narrative for non-medical readers, supported by full references to satisfy the medically qualified.

Progress in medicine has always been international. As will be seen, a major contribution to progress in surgery was assembled in Scotland during the reign of Queen Victoria.

Acknowledgements

I am grateful to Dr Iain Levack, anaesthetist and editor, who fifteen years ago invited me to review the practice of surgery in Aberdeen during the nineteenth century for the Infirmary Centenary book. This introduced me to surgeons here and elsewhere in Scotland who had had remarkably interesting careers. In this study I was helped by Mr Alexander Adam, Librarian of the Aberdeen Medico-Chirurgical Society, and I am very much indebted to him for his judgement and continuing interest during the writing of this book. I have been given the most willing assistance by a number of librarians – Wendy Pirie and her colleagues in the Medical School Library of the University of Aberdeen; James Beaton, the Librarian of the Royal College of Physicians and Surgeons of Glasgow; Marianne Smith in the Library of the Royal College of Surgeons of Edinburgh; the staff of the Library of the British Medical Association, with their knowledgeable and quick response to requests for reprints and the loan of books; Donald Orrock and Laura Adam of the Medical School Library of the University of Dundee; and the staff of the Cults branch of Aberdeen Public Libraries. Jackie Fiddes has provided willing and expert secretarial services. I am glad to acknowledge the expert help offered by Bruce Mirrilees and the staff of the Photographic Studio of the Department of Medical Illustration of the University of Aberdeen.

A generous grant towards the illustrations has been made from the Endowments Fund of the Grampian University Hospitals NHS Trust.

The role of a partner during the gestation period of a book is not easy. Margaret, my wife, has been a continuing source of encouragement, a valued critic of style, and a shrewd judge, on behalf of non-surgical readers, of the clarity of the text. It is a particular pleasure to dedicate this book to her.

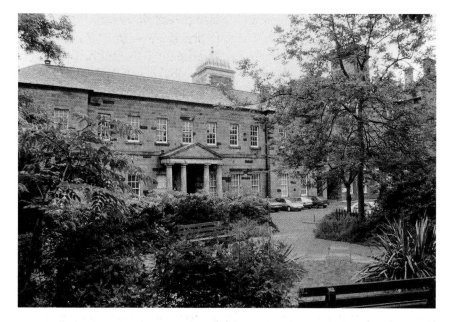

Fig. 1.1. The Surgical Hospital of the Royal Infirmary of Edinburgh from 1832 to 1879, which lies at the foot of Infirmary Street. Today its appearance is outwardly unchanged. Here James Syme and then Joseph Lister worked as Professors of Surgery. (P.F.J.)

CHAPTER ONE

Surgery before Anaesthesia and Antisepsis, 1837–1845

There remain two hospital buildings in Scotland which can stir memories of surgery as it was practised in the 1840s – one is in Edinburgh, the other in Aberdeen. Visitors walking up South Bridge in Edinburgh to visit Robert Adam's imposing 1780 building for the University can easily miss the narrow thoroughfare just opposite, named Infirmary Street. There is now no sign of the old building of the Royal Infirmary, which stood on the southern side of the street until the new Infirmary building opened on Lauriston Place in 1879. However, half-hidden at the foot of the street there is a low stone building, which was originally the Royal High School. When, in 1829, the School moved to Calton Hill, this building was bought by the Managers of the Infirmary, renovated, and a surgical amphitheatre built behind it to seat 400 students. It was reopened in 1832 as the Surgical Hospital of the Infirmary.[1]

Today, the outward appearance of the building is remarkably unchanged and one can stand in its forecourt and imagine some of its past visitors. From 1833, when he became the Professor of Surgery in the University, James Syme used to drive up to the portico at midday in his gig. Escorted by his house surgeon, he would go to his room, which can still be seen at the turn of the main staircase, and there greet visitors and interview patients, before moving on to the amphitheatre to lecture and then to operate.

5

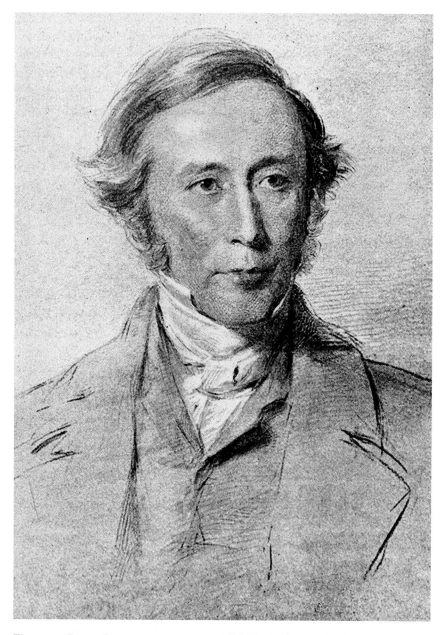

Fig. 1.2. James Syme as a young man. (McKay, W.J.S., *Lawson Tait*, London, 1922: 505)

Syme had graduated in 1821, at the age of 21, and served as a resident in the Infirmary, where he soon showed his characteristic independence of thought by declining to bleed patients who were already losing blood through haemorrhage.[2] He then taught anatomy with Robert Liston, who was five years his senior, and in 1822 he spent some eighteen months in Paris. There his anatomical knowledge benefited from the generous facilities for dissection. He attended many clinics and found the quality of the work of the Paris surgeons superior to what he had watched during his training. In particular he studied under Jacques Lisfranc who, in the course of a year, used 1,000 cadavers as he taught the techniques of the different amputations.[3]

Returning to Edinburgh in 1823 Syme passed the Fellowship examination of the Royal College of Surgeons. Even so, in September 1823, only two years after graduating, it is remarkable that Syme felt sufficiently experienced to tackle so major an operation as amputation through the hip joint (even allowing for the fact that this was known as Lisfranc's amputation, and that Syme had therefore had considerable experience on the cadaver under the direction of Lisfranc himself in Paris). The patient, William Fraser, was a youth who in 1821 was 17 years old, and had come to Syme with a hard tense painful swelling of the whole of the left thigh.[4] There was a sinus going down to bare bone near the knee, where an abscess had been drained, so this was probably a case of chronic osteomyelitis of the femur (this remained a condition quite familiar to surgeons until the advent of penicillin in the 1940s provided for the first time a treatment which arrested osteomyelitis at its acute stage). In 1821 no effective treatment could be offered and the patient naturally shrank from operation.

Syme called in to see William once or twice each week for about one year, and then lost sight of him until, in August 1823, Syme met William's father in the street, and learned that he was now determined on operation. When Syme, with Liston, saw William he had suffered many more abscesses and been confined to bed for two years: he was emaciated and got little sleep because of the constant severe pain. The swelling was larger and now extended to within an inch of the greater trochanter. 'A profound glairy discharge was poured out from many openings, he was feverish, and the pulse was small and very rapid.' After careful debate Syme and Liston could see no alternative, if the operation was to be carried out through healthy tissue, to amputation through the hip joint.

It is not known where the operation took place, but they proceeded on 2 September. The leg was held away from the table by an assistant, Liston compressed the femoral artery, and Syme took a knife one foot in length and, with an encircling sweep, he fashioned skin flaps, cut down through the tissues, and the leg was disarticulated at the hip joint and removed – a result taking 'at the most a minute' to achieve.

> Had it not been for thorough seasoning in scenes of dreadful haemorrhage, I certainly should have been startled. It seemed indeed, at first sight, as if the vessels which supplied so many large and crossing jets of arterial blood could never all be closed. We did not spend much time admiring the alarming spectacle. A single instant was sufficient to convince us that the patient's safety required all our expedition and, in a few minutes, haemorrhage was effectively restrained by the application of 10 or 12 ligatures.

The skin flaps were brought together with five or six stitches and roller bandages applied around the body and the stump. 'Then we lifted into bed the patient, who was wonderfully little exhausted.'[5]

In the evening the patient complained of much pain in the wound, which was found to be bulging – two sutures were removed and much blood clot evacuated, with immediate relief. He was seen at midnight, when he was very low and cold, and the pulse almost imperceptible, but next day he was a little stronger, beef tea was taken and morphia given four-hourly. By 4 September the lad was visibly easier, he slept well and by the twelfth day the wound was healing, and at one month progress was good. It was a deep disappointment that ascitic fluid then began to accumulate, weakness became progressive, and William died some eight weeks after operation. The post-mortem appearances suggested that he succumbed to amyloid disease.

What is hard to believe is that an operation of this magnitude could be tolerated, with no anaesthesia, and with the profound shock which must have been caused by the pain and haemorrhage. Moreover, there were no supportive measures such as would now be regarded as essential. Considering the fact that the instruments and the hands of the operators would just be washed, that the hands of the surgeons were constantly covering the wound to control bleeding whilst ligatures were applied, and that their operating clothes were usually covered in old blood, it is remarkable that the patient escaped a severe wound infection.

Syme, in his account of this operation, wrote: 'I am no advocate of operations whose only interest is their danger – and assuredly regard the knife at all times as a great, though too often necessary, evil'.[6] The surgeon of those days required a considerable collection of attributes. He needed good judgment, with a sympathetic assessment of the patient, to decide when the degree of distress and danger presented by the pathology was greater than the very real distress and danger intrinsic in the operation. He had to possess a combination of boldness and delicacy of touch, based on a comprehensive knowledge of anatomy, to enable him to operate at speed, in indifferent light, while knowing precisely where he was working, and the structures he must next meet or avoid. The strain of working in these conditions must have been great: John Abernethy was a distinguished London surgeon of the eighteenth century and his assistant described how 'he had seen him after a big operation with tears in his eyes, lamenting the possible failure of what he had just been compelled to do by dire necessity and surgical rule'.[7]

At this time Syme's major source of income came from lectures and tutorials in anatomy and surgery. Extra-mural classes, unconnected with the University, were a feature of Edinburgh medical teaching over many years, and students would pay to attend because they were well-run by keen but impecunious young surgeons.

In 1829, at the age of 30, Syme took a considerable risk, with borrowed money, when he opened his own small hospital in a disused town house – Minto House. By then his reputation was sufficient to attract patients, and there were young graduates who would subscribe apprenticeship fees for the privilege of assisting Syme. There were also many students who would pay to attend the practice of the hospital. By a small margin this income enabled Syme to keep the hospital afloat, and to treat many poor patients without payment. For over four years, Syme published a quarterly clinical report, which included many case histories. The 24 beds were always full, and some 40 students regularly attended. At that time Syme was short, slim and vigorous, his speech clear and concise, his personality rather quiet and solemn. He did tend to believe that his own views were the only correct ones, and so was often drawn into controversy. Nevertheless, friends and patients knew that, though he did not easily express gentler emotions, he had deep sympathies, and those who knew him best held him in great respect and affection.[8]

Syme had established something of a reputation for his skill in amputation, but he was also a leading advocate of more conservative measures. Then, and for a further one hundred years until the pasteurisation of milk became general, bone and joint tuberculosis was to remain common, especially among young people, and Syme showed that for many patients excision of the affected joint was much preferable to amputation. He particularly practised this on the elbow joint, thus preserving a useful hand.

By 1832 he felt that he had accumulated sufficient experience to write a book on the *Principles of Surgery*, which was unusual for being written in plain simple English, clearly founded on a wide personal experience, and the application of a few broad, safe, general principles. It was based on his lectures to students and was well received, going into several editions.

In 1833 the Chair of Clinical Surgery in the University became vacant, and Syme was appointed. The appointment meant that, though he was only classed as Assistant Surgeon to the Royal Infirmary, he had charge of 30 beds in the Surgical Hospital, with life tenure. Whilst still a young man, Syme had established himself in Scotland, and further afield, as a surgeon of great promise.

In the second half of the eighteenth century the streets of Edinburgh and Aberdeen still followed the haphazard pattern of

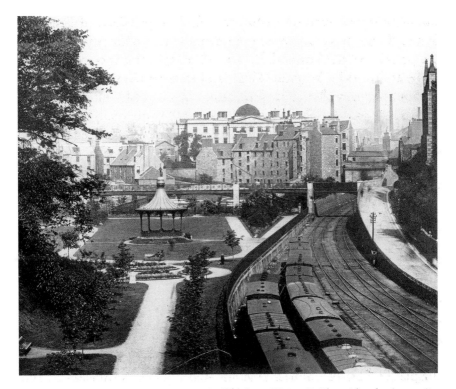

Fig. 1.3. The view of the Denburn Valley from Union Bridge, Aberdeen, as seen around 1880. The 1842 building of the Royal Infirmary lies on the horizon. The Den Burn was covered when the railway was extended to the north in 1867. The Gardens replaced bleaching greens when they were laid out in 1877. (Aberdeen Library and Information Services)

the Middle Ages, but by then both cities were expanding, and both embarked on major schemes of town-planning. From the 1770s, the New Town in Edinburgh was taking shape, and the North and South Bridge schemes allowed extension of the city to the south. In Aberdeen the ambitious Union Street project was conceived and adopted. The road from the south into the city was little more than a country lane and, stimulated by the Roads Commissioners, the City Council decided to lay out a straight, broad street, one mile long, running to the south. This involved the demolition of houses, the removal of a hill, and the bridging of the wide Denburn valley.[9] Thomas Fletcher, advised by Thomas

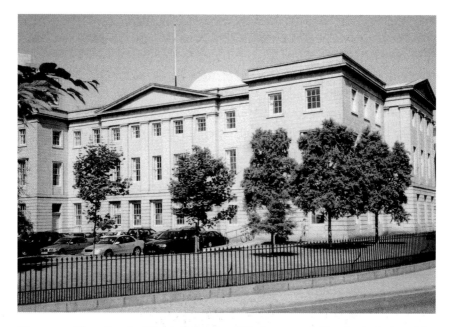

Fig. 1.4. The 1842 building of the Royal Infirmary of Aberdeen, designed by Archibald Simpson, as it appears today. The only operating theatre lay beneath the dome. (P.F.J.)

Telford, designed the bridge – a handsome stone single-elliptical arch, which was built between 1802 and 1805. The approach of Union Street to the bridge had to be carried on a series of arches, and the whole enterprise nearly bankrupted the city, but gradually finances recovered. Then the architects Archibald Simpson and John Smith, natives of Aberdeen, were able to design some of the handsome buildings which still grace Union Street.

In 1840 Aberdeen was a modest but busy town, with a growing population of about 60,000 (about one-quarter of the present size). In its shipyards the forerunners of the tea clippers such as the *Thermopylae* were being built for the races to China. There were active textile and papermaking industries, and the invention in the 1830s of machinery for the dressing and polishing of granite had given a great impetus to the exploitation of the local stone: most of nineteenth-century Aberdeen was to be built of it, and it enjoyed a ready market both nationally and internationally. Already some handsome buildings had come from Simpson's drawing board

– the Royal Infirmary, the Athenaeum, the Assembly Rooms, and the elegant townhouses in Bon Accord Square and Crescent. However, their civilised frontage hid primitive living conditions. One inhabitant recalled that although the houses had an 'ample entrance hall and staircase, and spacious rooms … there was no bathroom, no hot water in the kitchen and no sewer – the sewage passed into cesspools in the sunk area at the rear, closed by unsealed flagstones'.[10]

If a visitor in 1840 had chosen to pause on Union Bridge (fig. 1.3), the strong smell from the Denburn below – which was described as 'an open cesspool'[11] – would have spoilt the view. Beyond the bleaching greens beside the Denburn, which served the nearby cotton mills, lay Black's Buildings, a grim row

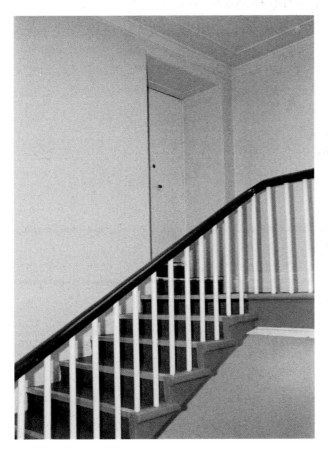

Fig. 1.5. At the top of the main staircase lies this narrow door, which was the only entry to the operating amphitheatre. Patients for operation walked up the stairs: on their return journey the patient was carried on a blanket, held at the corners by four students. (P.F.J.)

of tenements where families lived ten to a room, on six floors: these were damp and cold in winter and unbearably smelly and verminous when it was warm, with only a communal midden in the backyard, all water having to be carried up from the Well of Spa, some 50 yards away.

Just beyond these slums lay the newly opened Simpson pavilion of the Royal Infirmary, and here conditions in the new wards were not, in many ways, very much better. At the time of admission the patients, mostly poor folk, recommended by their parishes, were dirty, because the available means of bathing and the washing of clothes were primitive. Some patients in surgical wards suffered from typhus, and in 1863 the Matron died of the disease.[12] Surgical patients were rarely washed and Florence Nightingale, writing in 1854 in London, observed: 'nurses did not as a general rule wash patients, and they could never wash their feet. It was common practice to put a new patient into the sheets used by the last occupant, and mattresses were generally sodden.'[13] There was little encouragement to maintain cleanliness. One surgeon, writing of his student days in the Simpson pavilion in the 1860s, recalls 'how the wards, even the very corridors, stank with the mawkish manna-like odour of suppuration', and hardly a 'single wound healed without festering and small wonder'.[14]

In these circumstances it is not surprising to find that few operations were performed. The Annual Reports show that during 1840–44 about 1,000 patients were admitted to surgical wards annually, but only some 80–120 operations, or two each week, were performed. Apart from incisions of abscesses, these were limited to unavoidable procedures – amputations of limbs for compound fractures and tumours (and two for frostbite in servants), the occasional mastectomy for carcinoma, and each year 10–14 patients underwent perineal lithotomy for stone in the urinary bladder.[15]

Today the old Simpson building is quiet and clean, and it houses the school of physiotherapy, but one can still ascend the staircase to the top of the building, stand beside the narrow door which led into the only operating theatre, beneath the dome, and imagine the approach of a solemn procession – one can feel the terror and dread of the four-year-old boy with a bladder stone, or a woman facing

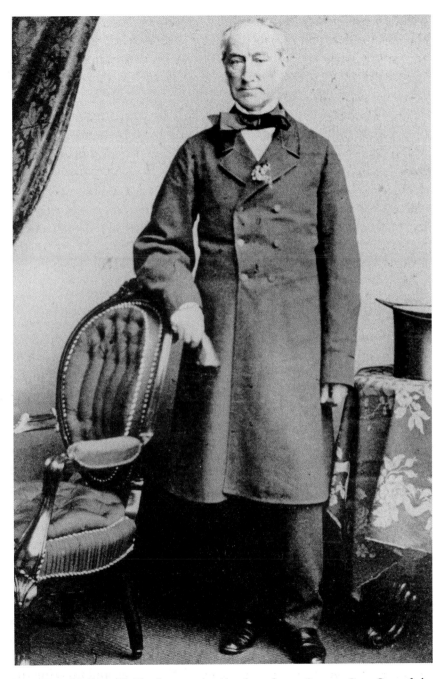

Fig. 1.6. William Keith, Surgeon in Aberdeen from 1833 to 1870. One of the first surgeons to write papers recording results in every patient – a forerunner of surgical audit. (Aberdeen Medico-Chirurgical Society)

mastectomy, as they were carried through the door into the noisy amphitheatre. The students, sitting in tiered rows, chattered and stared and demanded that their companions in the front row should remove their hats, while the patient was bound to the bloodstained wooden operating table. 'At the foot lay a wooden tray of sand, smelling of cats,' whilst on a shelf 'lay the instruments, open to anyone to handle. Suture needles were stuck into a jampot of rancid lard. There was no appliance for the washing of hands, and a dirty black frock coat covered with the dirt of years was donned by the surgeon.'[16] To the awful and immediate threat of unbearable pain there was, for both patient and surgeon, the very real prospect that post-operative sepsis would rob their suffering and his skill of a useful outcome. Although these circumstances seem to us so grim, to the people of 1840 they were in one respect not so different from the dirt and discomfort in which they lived – very dire for the poor and certainly smelly and potentially dangerous for the better-off, with no safe water supply, the only sanitary arrangements a hole in the ground, or a midden from which the contents were removed and carted out into the country.

In 1838 a vacancy arose on the staff of the Infirmary for a surgeon, and William Keith, aged 35, was appointed. Like most surgeons in those days, he would have learned his trade, as for any manual craft, by being bound apprentice for five years to a senior practitioner. As an apprentice he would act as assistant and dispenser: he would keep the surgery clean, make up medicines and roll pills, tend the leeches, keep the books, attend to dressings and draw some teeth, for nearly all surgeons spent most of their time and earned an income as general practitioners.[17] He would directly observe all forms of injury – fractures, dislocations, wounds and burns and scalds, the occasional strangulated hernia, retention of urine, hydroceles, and some problems in midwifery. At the limited number of operations performed the apprentice would act as assistant, but rarely if ever perform one himself, beyond opening the occasional abscess, or setting a fracture.[18] Later Keith passed the membership examination of the Royal College of Surgeons of England, and this suggests that he spent some time studying in London. (At that time the rules of the College were that at the end of his apprenticeship the young surgeon had to attend two courses of lectures and anatomical dissection, and then embark on a year of clinical experience at one of a limited number of teaching hospitals.)

We know little of Keith's life before 1838, but then he began a career, described in a series of papers, which reveals a remarkable character. From 1840 he had charge of 56 beds in the new Simpson building, to which 450–500 patients were admitted each year, although only 50–60 were actually operated on. In a paper published in 1844 Keith gave a detailed analysis of his first five years' experience of perineal lithotomy, or cutting for stone in the urinary bladder.[19] This condition was particularly common in cereal-growing areas of the country, and a majority of his patients were in fact farmers. It was remarkable for the intensity of the pain which patients – almost exclusively males – experienced on passing urine. This could become so severe and unrelenting that it exerted strong pressure on the surgeon to relieve these patients by lithotomy. (It must be remembered that, until X-rays became available at the end of the nineteenth century, the only way of positively identifying a stone in the bladder was from the history, and then by 'sounding' – passing a shaped, smooth metal staff down the urethra into the bladder and hearing and feeling the contact with a stone.)

In Keith's day the established operation for lithotomy was to approach the bladder from below, through the perineum – the area just behind the scrotum. This was a difficult operation. Keith reveals that he had never performed lithotomy before his appointment, but in preparation, 'I have borrowed ideas from every quarter, adopting what in my judgement was right in the practice of a variety of operators, and discarding what I thought wrong, and after all I find I make a close approximation to the plans of operation successfully practised by the father of English surgery, Cheselden, 100 years ago.' This care is shown particularly clearly in the detail with which Keith describes the correct position of the incision in the perineum, on which 'I, time after time, satisfied myself in the dissecting room'.[20]

Keith must also have been unusual in his day in the emphasis

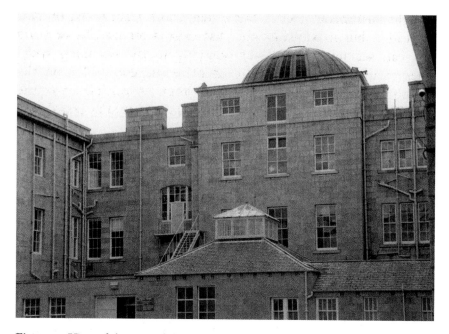

Fig. 1.7. View of the rear of the Simpson building. The only illumination for the operating theatre came from the skylight in the dome, and from the long north-facing window in the wall beneath it. (P.F.J.)

he laid on pre-operative preparation, especially directed to improvement in the health of the patient. This could take some time: he mentions how 'David Imray, aged 68: a poor, broken-down subject, having been recruited by good living for 9 weeks, was brought to the table'. Each of his patients spends an average of 60 days in hospital, of which '25 days are spent on previous preparation'. The average age of his patients was 56 years and many were 'wasted to a shadow, their strength quite exhausted by incessant suffering and want of sleep ... Strength is recruited by a generous diet and ample fluids. The inflamed bladder is treated by moderate but repeated leeching over the pubis.' Another and very different class presented in their fifties, 'fat and florid, in the highest state of plethora, and in the worst possible state for lithotomy'. They needed

a process of fining down by feeding them for 2–3 weeks on a

light farinaceous diet ... Some may think I am prolix on this head ... but in a disease that has existed for months or years I can see no necessity for hurrying to the operating table, especially as the kind and attentive surgeon will have the opportunity of securing the well-grounded confidence of the sufferer in his skill – desirable in every patient, but one almost essential to the success of lithotomy.[21]

The position of the patient on the operating table was of great importance. In 1840, with general anaesthesia as yet unavailable, five strong assistants were needed to control the inevitable struggles of the patient. He lay on his back, each leg bent up at the hip and held by an assistant, and flexed at the knee, with the hand bound to the ankle. This stretched the skin of the perineum, and the third assistant had the vital task of keeping the buttocks beyond the lower edge of the table by exerting strong downward pressure on the shoulders from the top of the table – the inevitable reaction of the patient to the pain of the operation was to withdraw up the table. The fourth assistant had the skilled job of passing the curved urethral staff up into the bladder, and holding it rigidly upright in position: this provided the essential guide to the surgeon for the route into the bladder. The fifth assistant successively passed the correct instrument into the hand of the surgeon, and generally assisted where required.

Keith then embarked on a detailed description of the siting of the incision in the perineum. Nowadays it is difficult for us to realise the awful tension which must have built up, both for the trussed-up patient and the surgeon, as they awaited the moment when an incision would be made in the perineum. Helped only by the light from the window behind him, the surgeon had to work at speed, yet with great attention to detail. The route was through the tissues of the perineum until the staff could be felt, identifying the position of the urethra. This revealed the way up to the bladder, which was then opened, and the stone removed with special forceps.

Keith then remarked: 'for beginners, let me warn that their trust must rest on a thorough knowledge of the parts concerned, a right apprehension of the principles that should control every step of the operation, and a calm calculatedness of mind, ready for any emergency' – advice as sound in the twenty-first century as in the middle of the nineteenth. Much useful detail is provided on the principles of extraction of the stone. This depended on the bladder neck being muscular, and so capable of being stretched by the forceps, to allow the extraction of a stone, but then being able to contract and heal.

At the end of the operation a tube was left in the bladder for several days: thereafter the leakage of urine along the track of the operation gradually diminished and usually ceased between ten and twenty days. Although the operating time was measured in minutes, 'there are few operations to which the adage *festina lente* does not apply. And to lithotomy it is especially suitable.'[22]

Then

> the comfort of the patient will depend on the unceasing attention of two experienced nurses, but his safety and progress rest, under God, on the surgeon's skill and care. For six hours he should never be above one hour at a time absent from the bedside, noticing the tube to keep it open, the colour and the quantity of urine, and resting satisfied in the head of haemorrhage. Then from the sixth to the thirtieth hour the surgeon should visit every 4 hours, and beyond that every 6 hours ... This should be continued for a week: it enables the surgeon to keep everything right, which is easier and safer than having to set them right. It also affords the opportunity for cheering the patient on – a matter of no light moment, the tendency to despond after this operation being very great.

Keith then commented on the fact that most patients expected to die, and it could be difficult to convince them that they would recover. For this reason,

> all condoling friends should be shut out for days after the operation ... let the surgeon minister to the mind as well as prescribe for the body; and while he rests on the blessing of God for success in the case, let him watch and strive as if the cure depended on his unaided efforts.[23]

Keith then considered aftercare: 'from the total silence on the subject in most practical works a beginner must conclude that there is little more to do: this is a great mistake. In old or feeble subjects the struggle for life only begins ... a diligent watch must be kept on the secretions, the tongue kept clean, soups allowed from the hour of the operation, and animal food from the third day. I do advocate more generous treatment as to diet after this and most other major operations. While there exists a call upon the constitution to heal up a great wound, do not keep the balance of life trembling from sheer want of food.' Keith found that to keep the patient reasonably dry the draw-sheet needed to be changed about eight times a day over the first eight days, and the buttocks required frequent treatment with spirit and prepared lard until the leakage of urine ceased.

The same attention to detail is seen in Keith's second paper, 'Hospital Statistics on Stone in the Bladder'.[24] (This is an impressive forerunner, by more than 150 years, of the attention only now being given to Surgical Audit.) 'Every case that presented to me for admission, whatever the age or state of health, was admitted and here accounted for. This I deem it necessary to state because (judging from my experience) if select cases only were to be operated upon, there need be few or no deaths after lithotomy or lithotrity.' Between March 1838 and March 1843 Keith admitted 43 patients with stone in the bladder: 4 were unfit for operation, 23 underwent lithotomy and 16 had lithotrity (crushing of smaller stones by an instrument passed along the urethra). All 23 patients who were lithotomised were male; 13 were over 60 years of age, but one was a boy of four and another a lad of 12 years. There were only 2 deaths among the 23 patients – one from spreading peritonitis, probably due to leakage of urine from an accidental tear high in the bladder. The other occurred in the four-year-old, William Kennedy from Nigg, who seems to have declined and died on the third day from blood loss and exhaustion. It is difficult not to feel that, at this age, the sheer strain and terror of admission to the crudities of an adult surgical ward, the anticipation and then reality of the operation, and afterwards the sight of six leeches applied to his lower abdomen to relieve pain, must have been a more desperate experience than he could sustain. For Keith, too, this operation must have been exceptionally stressful. Quite apart from his appreciation of the boy's feelings, he would have few instruments of the correct size, and to remove a stone which proved to be rather larger than a golf ball through the relatively tiny perineum would be a daunting task.

Each patient is documented by name, age and occupation (15 were farmers), with details of the first day on which urine was passed *per urethram*, the length of stay (always one month and often nearer two), and the size and weight of the stone.[25]

Keith's figure of two deaths in 23 lithotomised patients – which includes the first patients he ever operated on – is very creditable. Results generally depended very much on the skill of the individual surgeon, with Lisfranc in France reporting mortality rates for lithotomy mostly lying between 20% and 30%. Cheselden performed lithotomy on 213 patients at St Thomas' Hospital between 1727 and 1737, with 20 deaths (9.4%), which, for its time, long before antiseptic precautions, was a remarkable figure.[26] However, the majority of his patients were relatively young men, and only 14 were between 50 and 80 years of age, among whom 6 died; 19 of Keith's 23 patients came into this riskier age group, and there was one death, so his close study of Cheselden's methods had yielded an excellent result. In Dundee John Crichton enjoyed a strong reputation. In 1840 he was able to report 200 lithotomies with only 14 deaths – no details were provided, but this, too, was an outstanding record for its day.[27]

These two papers by Keith are remarkable in several ways. The candour with which he admits his inexperience, recounts such full details of the operation and then gives a complete account of his results is refreshing, but quite unusual. It is all very much in character, and the conclusion to his papers shows the source of the candour and sentiments of his writings.

Believing as I firmly do, that the issues of life and death are wholly in God's hands, I never fail urgently to implore his presence and blessing on every operation. From my bended knees I approach the operating table, the immediate effect of which is to impart to me a calmness that nothing can ruffle, a self-possession that has never been disconcerted, a steadiness of hand, and fertility of resource, that I thankfully acknowledge as gifts from God.

Nowadays this seems an unusual way to conclude an important surgical paper, and it might have aroused some comment at the time. However, 27 years later, Keith's friend Sir Henry Thompson, commented: 'He did it in singleness of heart, never dreaming that such simplicity could be doubted. I knew him well enough to be assured that it was the natural impulse of a trusting, childlike, and pious heart.'[28]

In the eighteenth and early nineteenth centuries surgery had in some ways reached, in a few hands, a level of technical skill based on manual dexterity and a most exact knowledge of anatomy, which has rarely been improved upon, and yet all surgeons were working in ways that had remained fundamentally unchanged for centuries. The practice of surgery continued to be, as the young Joseph Lister described it, 'this bloody and butcherly department of the healing art'.[29] All this was about to change.

CHAPTER TWO

The Arrival of General Anaesthesia, 1846–1860

During the 100 years before the 1840s, ideas had been circulating which promised hope of relief from the desperate pain inflicted during operations. Ether had been distilled in the sixteenth century and in 1744 Matthew Duncan, a surgeon in Manchester, England, recommended its occasional inhalation for the relief of chronic pain.[1] Then in 1799 Humphry Davy, 21 years old, prepared samples of nitrous oxide, and noticed that when he inhaled the gas it eased the pain he was suffering from a gumboil. With further experience he suggested that 'it may probably be used with advantage during surgical operations', although he did not pursue this further.[2]

Some years later these hints reached fulfilment in the lively atmosphere of the New England states of North America, where it became common in the 1820s and 1830s for young men to indulge in laughing gas (nitrous oxide) and ether frolics. It then became widely recognised that these agents sometimes produced a state of temporary insensibility. Itinerant lecturers were popular, and often gave demonstrations of the effects of laughing gas administered to members of the audience, among whom was Gardner Colton. In December 1844 he visited Hartford, Connecticut, where his lecture was attended by a local dentist, Horace Wells. Wells noticed that while some of Colton's subjects fell about the stage, and must have hurt themselves, yet they showed no signs of distress. At the time Wells was suffering from a septic wisdom tooth and he decided on a personal trial. He persuaded Colton to come to his surgery on the following day, to administer nitrous oxide while a fellow-dentist John Riggs extracted Wells's tooth. This test was successful and over the next month Wells and Riggs performed painless extractions on 15 patients under nitrous oxide anaesthesia.[3]

In the following year Wells moved to Boston, and this led to a meeting between Wells and John Warren, who was surgeon to the Massachusetts General Hospital. Their conversation resulted in Wells being invited in December 1845 to demonstrate nitrous oxide anaesthesia to Harvard medical students. A patient needing a tooth extraction agreed to be the subject. On this critical occasion Wells misjudged the depth of analgesia which he had achieved, and when the extraction began the patient complained loudly: the students barracked and the whole affair was a fiasco.[4] Although nitrous oxide has remained a valuable anaesthetic, it was for the time being overtaken by ether.

It is now largely forgotten that back in 1842 in Jefferson, a small town in Georgia, Dr Crawford Long found painful bruises on his body after participating in an ether frolic – he had no recollection of acquiring them. This led him to wonder if this property of ether inhalation could play a part in surgical operations.[5] He had a patient, Mr Venable, who had been delaying treatment of two lumps on his neck because he feared the pain of operation. When Long described to Venable his experience with ether, and suggested that he should try this for himself, Venable agreed and the operation took place on 30 March 1842. Ether was dropped onto the corner of a towel placed over the patient's face and he continued to inhale while one swelling (probably a sebaceous cyst) was painlessly removed. The other swelling was successfully removed a week later. Thus encouraged, Dr Long continued to use ether anaesthesia as cases arose in his country practice, and over the years he successfully performed eight mastectomies, and an amputation through the thigh. He also eased the course of five difficult obstetric deliveries with intermittent ether administration.[6]

Working in the far South, Long may not have heard of the Boston trials of 1846, and although his skills were well recognised locally, it was not until December 1849 that he felt he had sufficient experience to make a report in the *Southern Medical Journal*.[7] By then his modest but pioneering experiences had been overtaken by events all over the world.

The unsuccessful demonstration of nitrous oxide anaesthesia by Wells in Boston in 1845 had been witnessed by William T. G. Morton, a dentist who had been a partner of Wells in Hartford, and by a chemist, Charles T. Jackson. In later discussions Jackson suggested to Morton that ether might prove a more suitable agent for surgical work. Morton proceeded to test ether inhalation on himself and two of his assistants – not altogether satisfactorily. On the evening of 30 September 1846, Morton went with an assistant to his surgery and commenced inhaling ether, gradually losing consciousness. When he came round he realised that he had been insensible for 7–8 minutes. Then by a remarkable chance, late in the evening, there came a knock on Morton's surgery door. 'I found a man with his face bound up who seemed to be suffering extremely. Doctor,' said he, 'I have a dreadful tooth but it is so sore that I cannot summon courage to have it pulled.'[8] Morton assured him that he could ease the pain, quickly anaesthetised the patient, Eben Frost, and then, with a lamp held high to illumine the mouth, 'the firmly rooted bicuspid' was extracted. The patient had remained motionless and appeared quite lifeless. Deeply concerned, Morton flung a glass of water in his face and to his relief Frost woke up.

Subsequently, Morton administered 37 anaesthetics for Henry J. Bigelow (1818–90), who was surgeon to the Massachusetts General Hospital and later became Professor of Surgery at Harvard University. (The father of H. J. Bigelow was Jacob Bigelow (1786–1871), Visiting Physician to the Hospital, an eminent botanist, and Professor of Materia Medica: both father and son were close observers of the following trials of ether anaesthesia.)

With the experience he had gained in these cases, and with the support of H. J. Bigelow, Morton decided that the next step must be a public demonstration of the properties of ether anaesthesia. It must have been with some hesitation that he approached John C. Warren, in view of the earlier unsuccessful demonstration of nitrous oxide anaesthesia in Warren's theatre, but once again Professor Warren agreed, and the trial was set to take place in the same operating theatre of the General Hospital.

The patient chosen for this operation was Edwin Abbott, a thin weakly printer, 20 years old, who presented in September 1846 with a swelling under the right mandible which he had had since birth.[9] This extended down into the neck and into the floor of the mouth, where it was compressible and purple in colour. On 16 October 1846 Abbott was brought into the theatre, where the atmosphere was tense. The tiered rows of the amphitheatre were thronged with students, and many of the staff had gathered round the operating table. Morton arrived a little late and flustered, but he spoke some reassuring words to Abbott, and introduced Eben Frost: he could tell Abbott of his own reassuring experience. Morton then brought up his apparatus, Abbott breathed in a mixture of ether and air from a spherical flask, and in a few minutes fell asleep. Warren made an incision over the swelling, 3–4 inches long, and 'disclosed a congerie of large veins and small arteries. A curved needle armed with a ligature was passed under the mass and a knot tied with considerable compression'.[10]

H. J. Bigelow watched the operation and said that 'the patient muttered as in a semiconscious state'.[11] However, this cannot have been very apparent because the operation on 16 October was immediately recognised by the assembled company as a remarkable occasion, and Warren commented: 'Gentlemen, this is no humbug.'[12]

But we know from a letter Morton addressed to *The Lancet* in June 1847 that he himself was not happy – 'my first application was but partially successful. I found that in the meantime I must procure some more perfect apparatus' – because on the following day he was due to anaesthetise another patient in the amphitheatre.[13]

The original apparatus, used on 16 October, consisted of a glass sphere, some 125 cm in diameter, with two circular ports on opposite sides. Through one port a sponge was inserted, and a hollow wooden spigot was placed in the other. The sponge was soaked with ether, and the patient inhaled through the spigot, thus drawing in air over the sponge. Morton describes how, 'late on the night of the 16th, I conversed with Dr A. A. Gould when he rendered me important service in arriving at a valvular system which allowed the patient to expel each breath to the atmosphere. I had these valves introduced into a glass globe next morning, before my next engagement – at eleven o'clock at the hospital – when the fate of my discovery was to be settled. When the hour came, I went almost with a feverish excitement to the hospital. [Most] surgeons, physicians and all were incredulous, so my position was a most trying one. But with my new apparatus I went before the doctors – gave the ether – when the second capital operation was performed, this time with perfect success.'[14]

We know from Dr Bigelow's letter that this operation on 17 October was for 'a fatty tumour of considerable size, removed by Dr Hayward from the arm of a woman near the deltoid muscle … the operation lasted 4 or 5 minutes … the patient professed to have felt no pain, and to have known nothing of the operation. No doubt, I think, existed in the minds of those who saw this operation that the unconsciousness was real.'[15]

Dr Bigelow goes on to describe in some detail four dental patients, personally observed over the space of an hour, who had an extraction under ether anaesthesia administered by Dr Morton: all subsequently declared themselves quite unaware of any painful sensation. It is clear that at this early stage of the development of anaesthesia there was little attempt to prolong the length of administration. In those days of speedy operations this still offered great relief for two of the most common operations – extraction of teeth and the amputation of limbs. This was a momentous step forward for the surgery of the time, and many were involved in the early trials. However, it is due to the enterprise, courage and determination of one man – William Morton – that the vital early trials were conducted in public, in the presence of critical witnesses. These were occasions when he knew that it was his reputation alone which was at stake, and it must have required some resolution to carry on.

One of the remarkable features of these events in Boston, towards the end of 1846, was the speed at which news of the existence of ether anaesthesia spread to other countries. Here the advocacy of the Bigelows, father and son, played an important part. They seem to have spent several weeks observing the activities of Morton, and the final test seems to have been when Jacob Bigelow took his daughter Mary to Dr Morton's rooms in the middle of November: after a short ether anaesthetic she had a molar tooth painlessly removed.[16]

By the end of the month Jacob Bigelow was convinced that these results should be communicated to others, and his thoughts naturally turned to London, where Dr Francis Boott lived.* He was a fellow-American and a close friend of Bigelow over many years, during which they had shared a keen interest in botany. Jacob Bigelow enclosed with his letter of 28 November a copy of a lecture which his son, H. J. Bigelow, had delivered to the Boston Society for Medical Improvement on 10 November.[18] This package caught the next steamship to the United Kingdom – *The Acadia* – which left Boston on 3 December. It called at Halifax to take on passengers and coal and proceeded to Liverpool where it docked on 16 December. Dr Bigelow's package was delivered by the Royal Mail to Dr Boott's house, 24 Gower Street in London, on the following day, the 17th.[19]

Jacob Bigelow's letter of 28 November was brief, expressing 'strong belief in the power of ether, and its ability to relieve the pain of operative surgery', and quotes the favourable dental experience of his daughter.[20] Much more detail was provided in his son's report, which was enclosed.[21] These communications must have made a strong impression because Boott immediately made contact with his friend and neighbour, James Robinson, who was a dentist. Two days later, on 19 December, Robinson acted as both anaesthetist and dentist when he extracted 'a firmly fixed molar tooth' from a Miss Lonsdale under ether anaesthesia. This was done in the presence of his wife and daughters, as well as Boott himself.[22]

Boott had also lost no time in sharing the news with Robert

---

*   Boott had originally come to London as a youth, to promote his father's export business, but had gone on to study medicine in Edinburgh and to graduate MD in Edinburgh and LRCP in London in 1842. He employed his botanic interests as a Lecturer in Materia Medica, and in Physic. Dr Boott lived in Gower Street, and was involved in the foundation of University College and its Hospital, and he served for 30 years on the College Council. In this capacity he came in contact with Robert Liston, who in 1835 left Edinburgh to become Professor of Surgery in University College Hospital.[17]

Liston, and on his visit to University College Hospital that Saturday morning of 19 December, Liston met William Squire and told him of this great news from America of painless amputation. Squire was a medical student at the hospital, who had previously been introduced to Liston by Squire's uncle, who was Peter Squire, Pharmacist to the Queen and a friend of Liston. Liston had found William to be a keen student and he seems to have been adopted as temporary anaesthetist. Together they visited Mr Robinson and saw several people anaesthetised, ether being sprinkled on a sponge wrapped in a handkerchief which was held over the face.[23] This prompted them to find a better method of administration, and here Peter Squire became closely involved. He used the conical flask of a Nooth's apparatus, inserting a glass funnel into its neck: to the side-passage of the flask he attached a flexible tube into which was fitted a one-way valve and a facepiece. A sponge soaked in ether was placed in the funnel and then, with the facepiece applied over nose and mouth, the patient drew ether vapour mixed with air through the apparatus: the valve ensured that expired air was expelled to the exterior.[24] In experiments conducted by Liston, which included the administration of ether to William Squire, it was found best to surround the facepiece with a towel and to graduate the amount of ether taken in by placing the facepiece over or close to the mouth.

These trials continued on Sunday 20 December, as Liston 'looked into every detail for himself before arranging for the operation next day under ether'.[25] Messages were sent widely to members of the staff of University College Hospital, and other interested surgeons and medical editors were invited to attend, including Mr Robinson, the dentist. It is understandable that Liston should take such pains over these preliminaries: he was tall, with exceptionally large and powerful hands, and a deserved reputation as a skilful and remarkably speedy surgeon, which he guarded with some care. His temper was short and he would not be prepared to face a public humiliation, but he was also noted for his kindness to his patients, and had several unique techniques for minimising the pain of an operation, and would be careful to avoid raising false hopes over the potential of ether as an anaesthetic.[26]

The patient chosen for the demonstration was Frederick Churchill, a butler from Harley Street, a wasted pale-faced man with strumous (?tuberculous) disease of the left knee joint, with copious suppuration. He suffered much pain, which allowed little sleep, but had been too fearful of the pain of an operation to consent to it. However, when Liston offered him the chance of an operation without pain Churchill readily gave his consent. This took place on Monday 21 December 1846, at 2 p.m., in the amphitheatre of the hospital, in the presence of the Professors of Clinical Surgery and of Medicine, together with a large assembly of staff and students.[27] 'In a short address Liston spoke of the letter from America, of the advantages to be hoped from anaesthesia, of the weak condition of the patient, hardly able to sustain the operation without this expected aid, and asking the forbearance and quietude of all present.'[28] The patient was brought in by

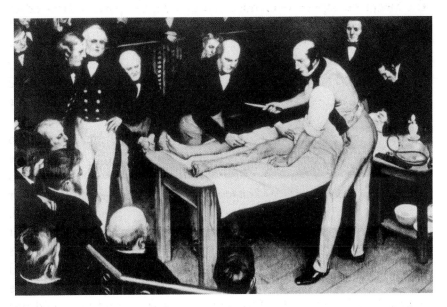

Fig. 2.1. An artist's reconstruction of the first demonstration of ether anaesthesia in Europe, which took place on Monday 21 December 1846. Robert Liston is about to amputate the left leg of Frederick Churchill. William Squire, the student anaesthetist (extreme right), holds the mask of the anaesthetic apparatus over Churchill's face, connected to the modified Nooth's bottle on the table through a length of tubing. Joseph Lister is standing second from the left. (UCL Art Collections, University College, London)

the house surgeon and positioned on the table. William Squire had his anaesthetic apparatus arranged on a small table and he spoke reassuringly to the patient, whose face was then covered with a handkerchief. The facepiece was introduced under this and the patient was asked to breathe deeply: the ether was taken easily and soon the breathing was deep and regular, and when unconsciousness was complete no more ether was given. Mr Squire said 'He is quite ready now, sir', and with that the limb was removed by Liston with his long amputation knife and the saw in 28 seconds. Arterial bleeding was secured with ligatures, and wetted lint placed between the flaps, which were then sutured together.

At this point the patient awoke and spoke, saying 'take me away, I can't have it off', and then he was lifted up to see the dressing – 'The expressive smile of surprise and delight with which he looked around is deeply impressed on my memory.'[29] Liston made his famous remark: 'this Yankee dodge, gentlemen, beats mesmerism hollow'.

Following the operation 'a marked change for the better in the patient's condition began at once, and led without interruption to a good recovery'. Squire goes on to make the just observation that 'the care and precautions taken in private under Liston's observation had much to do with the success of this first public trial of anaesthesia by ether, with the wide use it soon obtained, and with the strong conviction Liston formed of its very great importance.'[30] It is also surely fair to express appreciation of the role of William Squire who, though only a medical student, carried a major responsibility, and had so quickly learned the art of giving an ether anaesthetic. Within a few weeks Squire returned to his studies. (It was only in 1888 that he decided to record these very detailed memories – some 42 years after the event.)

During the evening of 21 December Liston wrote to Dr Boott (who could not attend earlier in the day), reporting the successful operation and observing that 'it is a very great matter to be able thus to destroy sensibility to such an extent, without apparently any bad result. It is a fine thing for operating surgeons, and I thank you most sincerely for the early information you were so kind as to give me of it.'[31] Then on 23 December Liston wrote

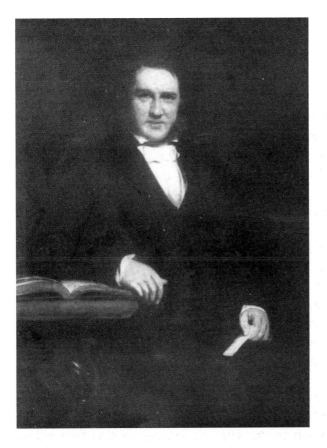

Fig. 2.2. Professor James Young Simpson, aged about 40. Simpson was only 28 when he was appointed Professor of Midwifery in 1840. He was 35 years old when in 1847 he demonstrated the properties of chloroform. (Turner, *Story of a Great Hospital*: 168)

to his friend James Miller, Professor of Surgery in Edinburgh, telling him of the successful operation on the 21st, and describing the apparatus devised by Squire for ether administration. Almost certainly Miller passed this letter to his neighbour James Young Simpson, the Professor of Obstetrics, who would be quick to recognise its significance. Indeed, Simpson must have left for London promptly, for Christmas found him spending the day with Liston, and doubtless hearing all the details of the recent trials of ether.[32]

In Edinburgh the first use of ether was on 9 January 1847, when the senior surgeon in the Royal Infirmary, James Duncan, performed a mid-thigh amputation on a young man who had an unhealed fracture of the femur. On 17 January Professor Miller operated under ether anaesthesia and removed a sequestrum from an unhealed compound fracture of the femur, using a Squire's apparatus which had been sent up from London by Liston.[33]

Two days later Simpson gave ether to a mother who was having a difficult delivery on account of a deformed pelvis: craniotomy was required to deliver a dead child, but the mother suffered no pain and subsequently did well. This is the first record of an anaesthetic being administered in obstetric practice, and thereafter Simpson regularly used ether at difficult deliveries, and went on to use it to ease normal deliveries – a completely new departure which aroused great controversy.

Ether anaesthesia rapidly became established in Scotland, although Syme did not at first find it an easy agent to use – probably he was rather too impatient to allow it to take full effect before commencing the operation. However, by August 1847 he had successfully adopted it.

Recently the record of a very early use of ether anaesthesia in Scotland, in unusual circumstances, has been described.[34] When the *Acadia* docked in Liverpool on 16 December, the ship's surgeon, Dr William Fraser, came ashore in order to spend Christmas with his recently widowed mother, who lived in Dumfries. When in early December the *Acadia* was docked in Boston, Fraser had apparently seen ether used and been suitably impressed. He travelled from Liverpool to Annan by steam packet and arrived home in Dumfries on 18 December. On that day or the next Fraser met an old school friend, Dr William Scott, who was a surgeon at the Dumfries Royal Infirmary, and naturally told him of his experiences in Boston. This only became public when, 26 years later, Dr Scott wrote a letter to *The Lancet* responding to an item in the previous issue.[35] This had stated that 'Liston was the first person to exhibit ether in this country.' Scott's reply to this claim said – 'I beg to state that I have a prior claim ... as I exhibited ether on 19 December 1846 to a patient in the Dumfries and Galloway Royal Infirmary ... I received my information relative to the anaesthetic properties of ether from the late Dr Fraser, surgeon of the Cunard steamer which brought the important news. I operated within 48 hours of the discovery being brought to this country.' Unfortunately there is no note of the operation performed, or of the patient's name, nor is there any entry in the records of the hospital, so this account compares unfavourably with the careful preparations of Liston and Squires for their public demonstration two days later. Subsequently James Simpson investigated this claim, and satisfied himself that it should be upheld.[36]

The news of the transformation of surgical practice which could be achieved through general anaesthesia spread rapidly. On 10 February 1847 *The Aberdeen Journal* reported that Dr Keith had administered ether to a boy of about 12 with scrofula (probably tuberculosis) of the ankle joint. The boy fell into a profound stupor, sufficient to allow an amputation to be easily and painlessly performed. Later, Dr Pirrie, Professor of Surgery, readily removed a tumour on the flank of a woman under the influence of ether; on waking she remarked 'what a sweet sleep, I am ready for operation!'[37]

In London Dr John Snow quickly became one of the first specialist anaesthetists, with appointments to University College, King's College and St George's Hospitals. Later in 1847 he wrote a book, *On the Inhalation of Ether*, and devised an apparatus to deliver a known concentration of ether in air to the patient. At the same time news of ether spread throughout Europe during January and February of 1847, then on to South Africa by April, and to Australia during May and June.[38]

At first the enormous benefit of unconsciousness during surgery gave ether a clear field, but it did have disadvantages – the vapour was strong and irritating, so inhalation was often uneasy, and its after-effects were quite long-lasting with troublesome nausea and vomiting. In home deliveries the ether bottle was heavy to carry, and in a sick room with an open fire its inflammability was a real hazard.

Consequently during 1847 the search for a kinder vapour went on, and probably the first to succeed was a Mr Furnell, who at the time was a medical student working as a pupil in the pharmacy of Mr Jacob Bell in London. Here the shelves carried many bottles containing aromatic substances and the curious Furnell, in the course of sampling their vapours, came across a bottle labelled 'chloric ether' (which is a solution of one part of chloroform in five parts of alcohol). Several chemists had isolated chloroform in the early 1830s, but Bell's source for this sample is not clear. The smell was pleasant, inhalation easy, and Furnell soon became drowsy: he told Mr Bell of this, who advised Furnell to go to St Bartholomew's Hospital and bring it to the notice of the surgeon, so in May 1847 he told Mr Holmes Coote (assistant to Mr William Lawrence) about his experience. Coote decided to test chloric ether that day, with very satisfactory results, and subsequently through the summer of 1847 a number of operations were conducted by Mr Lawrence under its influence. However, it was not until 1877 that Furnell, by then the Principal of the Madras Medical College, reported these facts,[39] and there is no doubt (readily acknowledged by Furnell) that it was James Young Simpson in Edinburgh who drew attention in 1847 to the qualities of chloroform.

During that year Simpson was testing a number of substances for their anaesthetic properties, using the simple but dangerous method of inhaling their vapours for himself, sometimes with serious effects. (Professor Miller in fact made a practice of calling at 52 Queen Street each morning to enquire after Simpson's health following the previous night's sampling.) Then, on a visit to Edinburgh in October 1847, David Waldie, who had been a fellow-student with Simpson, called on him. Waldie had moved to Liverpool, and there become a pharmacist.[40] They discussed potential anaesthetics, including 'chloric ether' (which Waldie knew to be a dilute solution of chloroform in alcohol), and Waldie promised Simpson that that he would prepare pure chloroform for him. However, in the meantime Waldie's workshop was burnt down, so Simpson looked elsewhere for supplies and despatched his assistant, Dr Matthews Duncan, to the laboratory of Dr William Gregory, Professor of Chemistry in the University of Edinburgh. Duncan collected a number of bottles containing 'respirable substances' and brought them back to Queen Street. Years later, in a letter to Dr Robert Christison in 1875, Duncan told how one morning he was casually sampling these vapours and took particular notice of chloroform, finding its scent so agreeable that he fell into a pleasant sleep for some minutes.[41] That evening Duncan reported his experience to Simpson, who thereupon embarked on a trial, with his two assistants (the other being Dr George Keith). Keith inhaled first and rapidly lost consciousness, and the other two then inhaled and fell to the floor. This was viewed with understandable alarm by Mrs Simpson and several of their children, but the experimenters, on recovery, were so satisfied with the results that they repeated their experiment several times, on to a late hour.[42] Simpson seems to have recognised immediately that chloroform offered many advantages over ether. Four days later, on 8 November, Simpson first used chloroform to assist the birth of a baby. On 12 November, at a demonstration in the Royal Infirmary, Simpson anaesthetised three patients on Professor Miller's operating list, the first being a boy of 4 who had a sequestrum involving most of the radius successfully removed: he was carried, still asleep, back to the ward where he awoke as from a refreshing doze. On 10 November 1847, at a meeting of the Edinburgh Medico-Chirurgical Society, Simpson read a paper on 'Insensibility to pain in surgical operations', and included the result of these trials.[43] The advantages which chloroform offered over ether were that a smaller dose was required, the breathing remained shorter and easier, it was cheap and portable, and it was not inflammable.

Chloroform rapidly displaced ether in Scottish surgical practice, and Simpson regularly used it in his obstetric work, although opposition in this field continued for some time. In Scotland the administration of an anaesthetic was at this time very much the responsibility of the surgeon. Joseph Lister, contributing the chapter 'On Anaesthetics' in successive editions of Holmes's *System of Surgery*, was able to state that 'Mr Syme has given chloroform about 5000 times without ever meeting a death', and Lister himself clearly wrote from long personal experience.[44] In Aberdeen Keith was convinced of the value of chloroform. He was able to anaesthetise a 3-year-old boy in his bed, bring him to the theatre, carry out a difficult perineal lithotomy, and return him to his bed where he awoke 'contented and happy'. Keith noted that lithotomy could now be done in boys, 'an operation he never deemed safe before the introduction of chloroform'.[45]

In London Dr John Snow,* who had established himself

---

* Dr Snow is rightly honoured for his work in a completely different field. He lived in Soho and witnessed several epidemics of cholera, with many

as a full-time anaesthetist, soon appreciated the advantages of
chloroform over ether, and went on to administer more than 4,000
anaesthetics, with only one possible death, and to write a detailed
account of its use. In 1853 Snow was asked by Queen Victoria's
Physician to provide chloroform analgesia during the delivery
of her eighth child, who was Prince Leopold. The Queen later
commented: 'Dr Snow gave that blessed chloroform and the effect
was soothing, quieting and delightful beyond measure.'[47] Since
1847 Simpson and other obstetricians had been dogged by strict
readers of Scripture, who believed it to be wrong to give relief
to women in labour, but this royal endorsement of chloroform
largely put an end to these complaints. Snow again gave his
services when the Queen was delivered of her last child, Princess
Beatrice, in 1857.

Soon, however, more cogent objections were offered. Quite
unpredictably the occasional patient died suddenly on the table,
and over time this happened often enough to generate a number
of enquiries. It became clear that although experienced users of
chloroform had evolved techniques which were consistently safe,
less practised anaesthetists were experiencing situations which led
to death. (John MacWilliam, Professor of Physiology in Aberdeen,
later showed in many animal experiments that chloroform had
a consistent toxic effect on the heart which was not shared by
ether. It produced cardiac dilatation, weakening of the heart and a
consequent fall in blood pressure: if dosage was misjudged, cardiac
arrest could occur.[48])

In the northern states of the USA ether remained the

---

deaths. It was clear to Snow that cholera was primarily an affliction of the
alimentary tract, and he strongly suspected the water supply as the source.
He is famous for removing the handle of the Broad Street pump in 1854,
but his best evidence was his study of the water companies. The Southwark
Water Company supplied unfiltered water taken from the sewage-laden
Thames at London Bridge: the Lambeth Company – whose pipes supplied
houses in the same streets as the Southwark – extracted water from the
relatively clean River Thames at Thames Ditton. Snow found that deaths
from cholera were 10 times more frequent in Southwark-supplied houses.
As soon as London's water was properly purified, outbreaks of cholera
ceased.[46]

anaesthetic of choice, and this was true in a number of centres in England, unlike Scotland where controlled use of chloroform was the rule. In 1872 Dr B.J.Jeffrey came over from Boston to demonstrate his techniques of ether administration in London. This visit, combined with a recognition that sudden death under ether anaesthesia was unheard of, led to a general return to the use of ether. This corresponded with the continuing rise in the number and complexity of operations following the adoption of antisepsis, and in the 1880s and 1890s with the growth in the number of abdominal operations (see fig. 7.6). These required good relaxation of the abdominal muscles, and it was relatively easy and safe to maintain deep ether anaesthesia without serious effects on the circulation or respiration.[49]

Chloroform continued to be used in obstetrics, and the ACE mixture (one part of alcohol, two parts of chloroform and three parts of ether), introduced in the 1860s, was for most of a century much favoured in general practice. (Soon after qualification in the 1940s the writer remembers acting as anaesthetist in the local cottage hospital, using ACE mixture dropped on a folded handkerchief held over the patient's mouth and nose.)

Overall, there was little change in anaesthetic techniques as the nineteenth century ended. For the first years of the twentieth century, ether, chloroform and nitrous oxide remained the only commonly used anaesthetics.

Joseph Lister

It was during this period, from 1846 to 1850, that Joseph Lister became a medical student. He plays so important a part in the remainder of this account that it is appropriate to introduce his story at this point.

Born in 1827 in Upton, Essex, the fourth child of Isabella and Joseph Jackson Lister, Joseph grew up in the quiet and studious atmosphere of their Quaker home. Although, with his sisters and brothers, there was plenty of activity, with games in the garden, riding, and long country walks with a close interest in natural history, no music was allowed in the house and there were no visits to theatres and concerts. The parents were devoted to their children but discipline was traditionally firm – when away at school J.J. Lister, aged 10, had received a letter from his own father John saying 'yr mother and I intended to have sent thee a plumb cake, had we had a better account, but shall now leave it to another time'.[50]

In the early nineteenth century Oxford and Cambridge did not admit Quakers, so many of them, J.J. Lister included, became established in business. Much of his leisure was devoted to the study of microscopy. It was he who, after mathematical computation and the polishing of his own lenses, developed the achromatic lens, which greatly enhanced the resolution of the optical microscope and led in 1832 to his election as a Fellow of the Royal Society of London.

Joseph soon caught his father's interests and became a keen naturalist, making fine pencil drawings of the skeletons of small animals and fish which he had prepared. Some early influence made him resolve to become a surgeon and at the age of 17, in 1844, he entered the newly founded University College in London: after three years in the Arts Faculty he graduated BA in 1847. The university had opened its own hospital in 1834 and there Lister went on to study anatomy and physiology. It was customary for students in their pre-clinical years to visit the wards of the hospital, and Lister himself has confirmed that he was among the audience who watched Liston perform his first operation under ether anaesthesia in December 1846.[51] While still a student, and with the encouragement of William Sharpey, Professor of Physiology, Lister used his early experience with the microscope to undertake a study of the muscular tissue of the iris of the eye, and was able to publish the first description of the constrictor and dilator fibres of the pupil. In 1851 Lister qualified and was house surgeon to the Professor of Surgery for 18 months. Then, remarkably early, he passed the examination for the Fellowship of the Royal College of Surgeons of England in December 1852. He went on to graduate MB of London University, with the Gold Medal in Surgery, in May 1853.

Operations at University College Hospital took place on a Wednesday, in the single operating amphitheatre, on an old wooden table lit by a single gas jet. The surgeons operated in

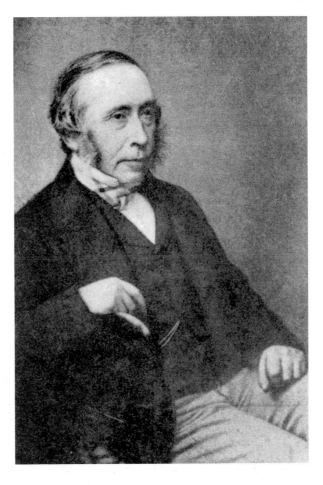

Fig. 2.3. James Syme, about the time that he and Lister first met. (Godlee, *Lord Lister*: 32)

order of seniority, watched by other members of the surgical staff. This gave little opportunity to trainees in surgery to gain practical experience, and Lister decided to visit other centres: Professor Sharpey advised him to go first to Edinburgh where Sharpey's close friend James Syme was Professor of Surgery.

By 1853 Syme was 54 years old, had held the Chair of Surgery for 20 years and had an international reputation. He was reputed never to waste a word, a drop of ink or an ounce of blood. When he lectured and operated in the amphitheatre of the Surgical Hospital 400 students would assemble. If operations were scheduled for a Sunday, the students would first attend Lady Yester's Church in Infirmary Street, but when they heard the

Infirmary bell announce the start of operations they thundered out of the gallery and raced down to the theatre: the preacher found it best to interrupt his sermon until silence returned.[52]

An observer in the forecourt of the Surgical Hospital one day in September 1853 might have seen an apprehensive visitor – Joseph Lister, aged 26 – walking towards the entrance portico (see fig. 1.1): perhaps he paused to ensure that Sharpey's letter of introduction was still in his pocket. His intention at that time was to spend a month with Syme and then move on to visit surgical clinics in Europe. He would hardly be reassured as he entered the dingy, smelly, crowded building and mounted the stairs to Syme's room. Syme was said to be taciturn and difficult, but he and Lister seem to have understood each other from the start: within days Lister could report to his father that he had been called from his bed at 5 a.m. to travel with Mr Syme to Dunblane, to serve as his assistant at an amputation through the shoulder joint. 'I had

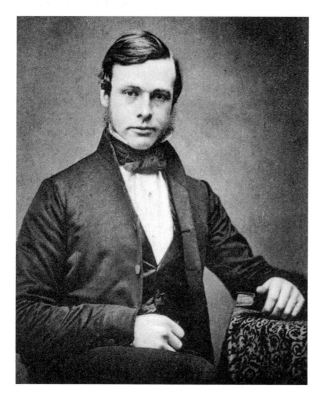

Fig. 2.4. Joseph Lister aged 26, at the time he first came to Edinburgh. (Godlee, *Lord Lister*: 42)

the honour of acting practically as the only assistant, who on such an occasion is a rather responsible officer.'[53]

Soon, Syme appointed Lister to be his supernumerary house surgeon, and all ideas of travelling in Europe were postponed. Lister was conscious of all he could learn working among the 200 surgical beds in the Infirmary, assisting Syme at every operation, taking notes and caring for the post-operative patients. This proved to be a turning-point in Lister's career, and at the end of 1853 he told his sister that he was resolved to pursue a career in 'this bloody and butcherly department of the healing art ... I am more and more delighted with my profession ... and Syme's kindness continues to flow steadily and if possible increasingly.'[54] This was very soon confirmed when early in 1854 Syme's resident house surgeon was called away, and failed to return. Lister was able to step into his position and remained in the post until January 1855. This made him responsible for the continuing supervision of Syme's patients, the teaching of his 12 student dressers, and the use of his own discretion over all patients admitted at night, including the performance of any necessary operations. For Lister to have carried this degree of responsibility for a year was invaluable experience.

Chloroform was then the anaesthetic of choice, so surgery was no longer quite so 'butcherly' as it certainly was before 1846, but the range of operations performed was still limited – mainly amputations, the occasional mastectomy and cutting for bladder stones – while speed was still considered a virtue. The risks of post-operative wound sepsis were as real as ever, and conditions in the wards remained primitive, with admissions more or less restricted to those who could not afford a doctor's visit. Many came from the grim closes of the High Street, so narrow that the sun never entered, where there was no running water or sanitation for the overcrowded rooms. The inhabitants naturally arrived in hospital unwashed and in dirty clothes, so the bed linen and surgical wounds soon became contaminated. 'By day two senior nurses staffed the 72 beds in the Surgical Hospital, and through long experience were highly skilled. However at night the wards were in the care of a changing and unreliable band of charwomen, not always sober. For any major postoperative case the student dressers of the firm organised themselves into four-hourly shifts, and kept strict watch over the progress of the patient.'[55]

Through 1854 and 1855 Lister kept notes of Syme's lectures and used these to provide *The Lancet* with weekly reports of the proceedings – 'the result of an acute and comprehensive mind working upon an experience of upwards of 30 years'. Usually two subjects were covered, arising from the diagnosis and treatment of patients who had presented in the wards.[56]

In March 1854 Britain had embarked on the Crimean War against Russia and in September Britain and France invaded the Crimean peninsula and laid siege to Sevastopol. Among the many medical volunteers was Dr Mackenzie, who was an Assistant Surgeon at the Royal Infirmary of Edinburgh, and Lecturer in Surgery at the College of Surgeons: it was thought likely that he would succeed Syme in the Chair of Surgery. He demonstrated his surgical skills at the Alma River battle in September, but this promising career ended abruptly when he succumbed – like many others in the Allied armies – to an epidemic of cholera. Lister was asked to take on Mackenzie's winter course of lectures.

In January 1855 Lister's time as Syme's resident ended. He continued to report Syme's lectures and moved into lodgings in Rutland Street. There he began a study of the early stages of inflammation, turning his microscope onto the web of the feet of frogs caught in Duddingston Loch. The frog was anaesthetised and the web of the foot fixed on the stage of the microscope, so that it could be examined with a low-power lens. This allowed study of one artery, with the web of capillaries into which it divided: then the reaction to a drop of very hot water, mustard and other irritants was studied. These sessions often extended far into the night, the work being pursued over the next two years. In April 1855 Lister was elected a Fellow of the Royal College of Surgeons of Edinburgh, which gave him the freedom to see private patients. He also rented a room alongside the Surgical Hospital where in November he would commence a course of lectures on the Principles and Practice of Surgery. Another matter also preoccupied him, for a growing attraction had been maturing between Lister and Syme's daughter, Agnes, and this culminated in July in their engagement.[57]

The experiments on inflammation continued, he prepared and delivered the course of lectures, saw the occasional private patient, and hunted for a house and furnishings. In April 1856 Agnes and Joseph were married, and departed on an enterprising continental journey to Germany, Austria and Italy. This must have been a much more enjoyable and fruitful expedition for Lister than the journey he had planned when he set out for Edinburgh in 1853.

The Listers' home was in Rutland Street, less than five minutes' walk from Princes Street Gardens, where Lister liked to walk before breakfast, planning lectures and the layout of papers. In October he was unanimously elected an Assistant Surgeon to the Royal Infirmary. In this position Lister found himself in charge of Syme's patients when he was away, and early in 1857 Lister wrote to his father about

> a very ticklish operation ... on a large tumour in the armpit. The theatre was again well filled, and though I felt a good deal before the operation, I lost all consciousness of the spectators during its performance. Just before the operation began I recollected that there was only one Spectator whom it was important to consider, one present alike in the operating theatre and the private room.[58]

One room in their house was set aside as a laboratory, and here Lister and Agnes would work over the microscope in the evenings, often continuing as before into the early hours. Agnes soon became an expert assistant and secretary, keeping the records and assisting in the writing of some 15 papers during 1857–1860, including the long paper on the early stages of inflammation which was read to the Royal Society of London. Such a record would be impressive today, but in Lister's day it was remarkable. Surgeons were men of action, and there was barely one who had a laboratory, with a microscope, in his house. Here Lister's upbringing, and the example and teaching of his father, were vital elements.

So was Lister's respect for John Hunter, the raw young man from Lanarkshire who in 1748 went to London to assist in the anatomy room of his brother William. In time, John became a skilful surgeon, and a great collector, which led him on to many investigations. It was Hunter's experiments on the arterial circulation in the horn of a stag which led him to the operation of high ligature of the superficial femoral artery in the thigh, to relieve popliteal aneurysm. His essential attitude was summed up in his aphorism – 'why ponder and speculate?: try the experiment'.[59]

Lister always kept an engraving of Hunter's portrait on the wall of his study: like Hunter, he was a scientific sceptic, with an unusual ability to devise the right experiment to solve a debatable matter. Each year he would urge his class to think for themselves – 'never let theories stand in the way of your own observations'.[60]

Increasingly Syme was leaving Lister in charge of his wards and the teaching, while remaining available for consultation – a great opportunity to consolidate experience. In August 1859 it became known that the Regius Professor of Surgery in the University of Glasgow was in poor health, and the search for a successor had begun. During his six years in Edinburgh Lister had built up an excellent reputation, combining clinical and operative skill with a popular style of lecturing and teaching: his modesty and transparent honesty were widely appreciated. Lister's record of experimental research and his published papers were exceptional, and it was only a few months later that he was elected a Fellow of the Royal Society of London. Though only 32 years old, Lister decided to apply for the Glasgow post, and in January 1860 he received a letter from the Home Secretary confirming his appointment to the Regius Chair. He was warmly congratulated by his colleagues and by the student body, and the Listers were left in no doubt that there was real regret over their departure.

They moved to Glasgow in May 1860, taking up residence at 17 Woodside Place, which lay in a pleasant Georgian terrace, recently built in the West End of the city. Kelvingrove Park lay a few minutes away, so once again Lister was well placed for his early morning walks. At the time of his appointment he had understood that he would soon be appointed a Surgeon to the Royal Infirmary, so he was surprised to find that he was expected to wait and apply for the next vacancy on the staff. Finding that

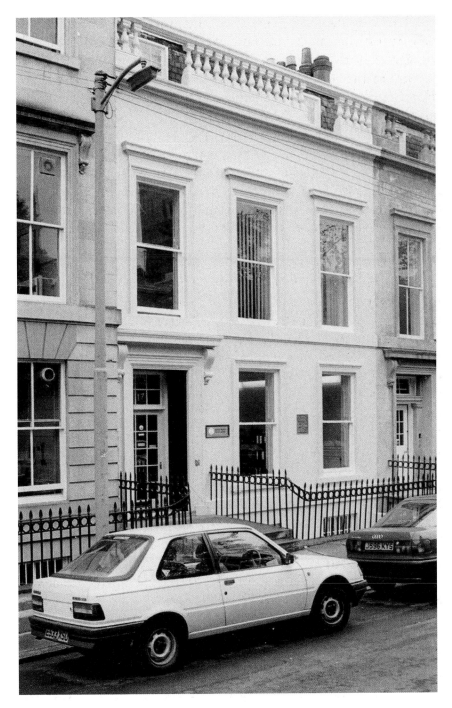

Fig. 2.5. 17 Woodside Place, the Listers' home in Glasgow. (P.F.J.)

the academic session had just begun, Lister decided to deliver a short summer course of lectures. These were given on the campus of the old University which, built in the sixteenth century, still lay in the old part of the city, on the High Street, close to the Royal Infirmary and surrounded by some of the most crowded closes and tenements in Glasgow.

The lecture theatre was dark, dusty and showing its age, so during the vacation the Listers had it redecorated, the desks were mended and they installed a proper blackboard. When the full winter course of lectures started, the students showed their approval of the renovations by removing their hats. At the end of his first address Lister spoke, characteristically, of the two great

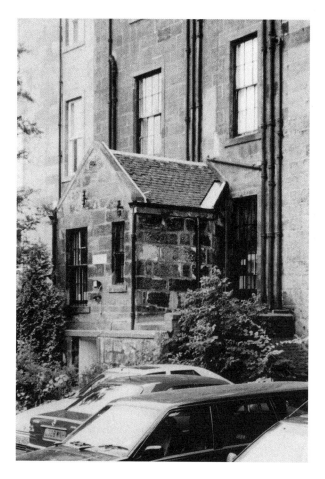

Fig. 2.6. The laboratory which Lister had built at the back of 17 Woodside Place. (P.F.J.)

requisites for the medical profession – 'First a warm and loving heart, and secondly, Truth in an earnest spirit'.[61] The young new professor was roundly applauded and soon the lectures were attracting a class of 182 enthusiastic students. Lister needed some encouragement because his first application to join the staff of the Infirmary was, remarkably, not successful. (When in the course of his canvass Lister told the Chairman of the Infirmary Board of Directors that he needed to illustrate theory with practical clinical teaching, he was told that the purpose of the institution was 'a curative one. It is not an educational one.'[62]) When the course of lectures ended, 161 members of the class signed a parchment signifying their approval, and offering the strongly expressed wish that Lister's application for a place on the staff of the Infirmary would be successful.

During this waiting time Lister built a small laboratory onto the back of his house. Although cars are now parked throughout the Woodlands Estate, its general appearance is little changed since Lister's time. 17 Woodside Place is now a busy office, but one can admire the handsome ceiling in what was the dining room, and stand in the old consulting room. Then there is a door which reveals the laboratory, with the wooden shelves designed by Lister fitting into awkward corners. Here he and Agnes collaborated over their experimental work, while he waited for the opportunity to work at the Infirmary. Below in the basement of the laboratory is the washhouse where Agnes cared for a calf for several days until experiments could be carried out. Finally, on 5 August 1861, they learned that Lister had been elected a Surgeon to the Royal Infirmary.

CHAPTER THREE

The Path towards Antisepsis, 1795–1865

Pioneers of a Revolution

Before going on to examine the steps which led Lister to ponder on Pasteur's researches, develop the antiseptic regime, and from there to work out the basis and details of *The Antiseptic Principle in the Practice of Surgery*, it is necessary to go back to a time when there was no knowledge of the existence of germs and micro-organisms. For centuries it had been evident that smallpox, syphilis, gonorrhoea and measles could spread from person to person, and were contagious diseases, but the responsible agent remained obscure. Most people, including the medically qualified, spoke of miasmas or 'bad air'. An Edinburgh medical dictionary of 1807 defined miasma as 'a particle of poison in a volatile state, borne on the wings of the atmosphere, and capable of attaching itself to an animal body so as to produce disease ... as in the case of contagion'.[1] Hence the wide use of fumigation of rooms, furniture and bedding during times of plague.

The study of puerperal fever by a few pioneers provided some hard facts which pointed the way forward. One of the first was Alexander Gordon, who was born in the Aberdeenshire parish of Peterculter in 1752, and who graduated MD in Aberdeen in 1778.[2] He served for some years as a naval surgeon, and then during 1785 he spent nine months in London, studying the practice of midwifery in the British Lying-in Hospital. Here, as happened in every maternity hospital, outbreaks of puerperal fever occurred. Two to three days after the delivery a mother would run a high fever and develop an offensive vaginal discharge which, in about one mother in four, progressed to a spreading peritonitis, bloodstream infection and death. There was no effective treatment, although subsequent study of the spread of puerperal fever led to useful preventative measures. It remained a serious and tragic complication of a natural process for another 140 years, and even in the early 1930s it still caused some 1,500–2,000 maternal deaths each year in England and Wales.[3]

In 1786 Gordon returned to Aberdeen as Physician to the City Dispensary – a general practice which included the care of many pregnant mothers in their homes, and the supervision of a number of midwives.[4] Here, during 1789–92, Gordon witnessed an epidemic of puerperal fever which appeared seemingly casually among his patients in their homes: finally 76 mothers were affected. It was Gordon's habit to keep notes on all the patients in the practice and later, as he listed the fever patients and the names of the 17 midwives who worked with him, he came to the conclusion that a case of puerperal fever only arose when the mother had been attended by a midwife (or himself) who had come from attendance on another patient who already had the fever. In the course of time he realised that he could 'venture to foretell what woman would be affected by the disease upon hearing by which midwife they were to be delivered – and in almost every instance my prediction was verified. I plainly perceived the channel by which it is propagated.' Gordon recognised that the open wound left in the uterus was the site of entry for 'a specific contagion or infection', which was not due to a 'noxious state of the atmosphere' because the pattern of spread of infection was demonstrably not random, occurring only after the visit of a carrier. 'With respect to the physical characters of the infection I have not been able to make any discovery, but I have evident proofs that every person who had been with a patient with puerperal fever became charged with an atmosphere of infection, which was communicated to every pregnant woman who came within its sphere.' Gordon went on to admit that 'it is a disagreeable declaration for me to mention that I myself was the means of carrying the infection to a great number of women'.[5]

Gordon made another important observation. He stated that

'Puerperal Fever is of the nature of Erysipelas, they are connected, and occurred in concomitant epidemics, kept pace together, and both ceased at the same time.' Erysipelas is an acute infection of the full thickness of the skin, occurring most often on the face. It spreads rapidly, with a characteristic raised edge. The shrewd observation of Gordon, often confirmed in later outbreaks, was explained 85 years later when the cause of puerperal fever and of erysipelas was shown to be infection by Group A *Streptococcus pyogenes.*

The passages quoted above are taken from a full report which Gordon published in London in 1795, entitled *A Treatise on the Epidemic of Puerperal Fever of Aberdeen.*[6] In this he included a table which gave details of each of the 76 women affected, and which included the names of the doctors and midwives concerned. We can now see that this was an error because it showed that some individual midwives were much more associated with spread of the contagion than others: naturally this caused great offence when the *Treatise* reached Aberdeen. Gordon's practice soon fell away and he found it expedient to return to service in the Navy. Within four years he had died from pulmonary tuberculosis, at the age of 47. His *Treatise* and his clear and practical conclusions seem to have attracted little notice; however, it was reprinted three times over the next 55 years, the last edition appearing in Philadelphia in 1842.

In the following year Oliver Wendell Holmes, a practitioner in Boston, USA, learned of the death of an obstetrician from septicaemia. During an autopsy on a patient who had died of puerperal fever, this friend sustained a cut on his finger. Following this injury, and before falling ill from spread of infection in the cut, he conducted several deliveries on patients, all of whom developed puerperal fever. Holmes, who later became Professor of Anatomy at Harvard and a well-known author, felt that this sad experience needed exploration, so he carried out a thorough review of the literature of that time, including Gordon's report. In a long paper entitled 'The contagiousness of puerperal fever', read to the Boston Society for Medical Improvement in February 1843, Holmes found that the weight of evidence was clear – that 'the disease known as puerperal fever is so far contagious as to be frequently carried from patient to patient by physicians and nurses'.[7] Holmes quoted one lecturer as saying: 'in my own family I had rather that those I esteemed most should be delivered, unaided, in a stable, by the manger-side, than that they should receive the best help, in the fairest apartment, but exposed to the vapours of this pitiless disease'. Holmes considered it obligatory that obstetricians should never take part in autopsies on fever patients, and once they had attended a patient with puerperal fever they must seriously consider whether they should expose another expectant mother to the risk of infection until 'some weeks' had elapsed. Perhaps because this specific warning was given without a clear idea of the cause of the infection, and because it came from a young and inexperienced physician, Holmes's strong advice was received with scepticism, and with direct opposition from the Professor of Obstetrics in Boston. Holmes commented sadly: 'behind the fearful array of published facts there lies a dark list of similar events, unwritten in the records of science, but long remembered by many a desolate fireside'.[8]

Three years later there came a major contribution to the debate from Dr Ignaz Semmelweiss who, from 1846, worked as assistant in the delivery wards of the main lying-in hospital in Vienna.[9] Mothers were admitted into one of two separate divisions, A being run by the obstetricians, who also taught the students, while Division B was solely in the care of female midwives. It was soon clear to Semmelweiss that the incidence of puerperal fever in Division A was some three times higher than it was in Division B. He argued that it was significant that doctors and students in Division A, who had often come from other wards and even the post-mortem room, did not always wash their hands before examining patients internally. So, in 1847 Semmelweiss instituted in Division A a strict routine of hand-washing and scrubbing, followed by a rinse in chlorine water, before any patient was examined. Within a month this was clearly having an effect, and it was found that the mortality rate in Division A (which was 10%) had come down to 3%, the same as in Division B. Although he did not know the real reason for unwashed hands being so dangerous, Semmelweiss spoke of the transmission of 'cadaveric particles'. He had made two major observations. He provided further proof of Gordon's finding that puerperal fever is an acquired infection transmitted by direct vaginal inoculation and, vitally, he had shown for the first time how, by practising antisepsis, cross-infection could to a large extent be prevented. Like Gordon and Holmes, Semmelweiss had his critics and, though strongly advised by his friends to publish his impressive results, he did not respond. Semmelweiss was an odd character, and he soon left Vienna for a post in his native Budapest, and only in 1861 did he publish a long and poorly organised report 500 pages long.[10] This seems to have had little effect, and even in Vienna the antiseptic routine did not long survive his departure. For many years Semmelweiss and his work seem to have been forgotten.

In 1850, J. Y. Simpson, the Professor of Obstetrics in Edinburgh, wrote a thoughtful paper on 'The analogy between puerperal fever and surgical fever'.[11] He observed that while the surgical patient had an external wound made by the surgeon's knife, 'in the puerperal patient we have a wound of the whole internal surface of the womb made by separation of the placenta'. Air can enter both these wounds 'and frequently they are apt to be followed by febrile and inflammatory reactions which we term surgical fever in the surgical patient, puerperal fever in the puerperal patient. In short, the two species of wounds are of the same pathological nature ... liable to be attended with the same pathological effects and complications.'[12]

Later, Simpson wrote that ' I have taught for the last 10 years that there exist, I believe, facts sufficient to prove that patients during labour have been and may be inoculated with a *materies morbi* capable of exciting puerperal fever, that this material is liable to be inoculated into the dilated and abraded maternal passages during delivery by the fingers of the attendant, and that thus [it is transferred] from one patient to another.'[13] Simpson then quotes the success of Semmelweiss in his insistence that his students should wash their hands in chlorine water. A year later in 1851 Simpson revealed that he 'had used for the same subject for years, daily (or often during the day), a solution of cyanide of potass' to cleanse his hands.[14] This suggests that Simpson preceded Simmelweiss in recognising the need to sterilise the hands of the accoucheur; however, if he made this a regular part of his practice he did not record his results. Credit must be given to both these individuals for their constructive thinking, but it was Semmelweiss who provided the first convincing demonstration of the potential of antisepsis in the prevention of an infection.

It is remarkable that more notice was not taken of these findings because the risk of death from puerperal fever among mothers delivered in maternity hospitals was very high, when compared with deliveries in the mother's home. In 1865 a report on Queen Charlotte's Hospital (the leading lying-in hospital in London) showed the death rate per 10,000 deliveries was 263, compared with mothers delivered, often in primitive circumstances, in their homes in the East End of London, for whom the figure was only 27.[15] Although general obstetric care in these hospitals was of a high standard, the existence of germs was not recognised, and so it was not realised that the bedding and the dust on the floors were heavily contaminated, and this, combined with imperfect hand-washing, meant that cross-infection among patients was common. Two years later, Lister's first papers on the potential of antisepsis were published. It took some time for this advance to be accepted in surgical circles, and it was only in the 1880s that obstetricians realised that Simpson's comments in 1850 on the similarity between surgical wounds and the puerperal uterus had been prophetic. The application of the antiseptic principle in surgical practice forecast how it could be used to prevent many cases of puerperal fever; when this was done the results were equally remarkable, and they spread rapidly round the world. In Boston, USA the Lying-In Hospital had to be closed for some weeks in 1879, 1880 and in 1883 because of the frequency of outbreaks of puerperal fever, and even after thorough fumigation the outbreaks continued. From 1884 Listerian reforms were introduced, including the sterilisation of instruments, handwashing in antiseptic before and after touching patients, washing of the external genitalia and use of sterilised sanitary towels. Previously, the mortality rate (per 10,000 births) had ranged between 450 and 550, but in 1884 it was 64 and in 1886 there were no deaths from sepsis.[16] Hospitals in London and Sweden reported similarly.

At this time the true cause of puerperal fever was becoming clear. As early as 1869 Coze and Feltz in Strasbourg found *microbes en chainettes* in the lochia of patients with puerperal fever. Doleris in a monograph in 1860 gave a full description of micrococci arranged in chains in the lochia, and Pasteur confirmed this, as did Ogston in Aberdeen. Doleris named these germs *micrococcus pyogenique*, a forerunner of the modern name of *streptococcus pyogenes*.[17]

Over the next fifty years obstetric care devoted special attention to the prevention of infection. During the 1920s and 1930s much was learned about the streptococcus and its many different strains and virulence. The work of Leonard and Dora Colebrook and Ronald Hare at Queen Charlotte's Hospital revealed an important and previously unsuspected source of transmission when they showed that a natural reservoir of streptococcal infection lay in the human nose and throat. Among the staff of the hospital, 5–10% were unwitting nasal carriers of potentially pathogenic streptococci, and this was also the case among ordinary families. It was clear that this could account for many unexplained epidemics. As a consequence the wearing of masks and of sterilised rubber gloves, with regular culture of nasal swabs among staff, was widely adopted, yet even when these precautions were strictly applied the virulence of some strains of streptococci meant that cases of puerperal fever still arose, and in severe cases the mortality rate was still about 25%.[18]

As it happened, the mid-1930s saw the start of a remarkable decade of development of chemotherapy, which has become so vital an element of medical care. Domagk in Germany had been working for some time, in the Bayer laboratories, on the possible value of chemical dyes in the treatment of bacterial infections. In 1935 he was testing a red dye, Prontosil, and found that it had a dramatic effect: mice, when inoculated with a virulent strain of streptococci, survived if given a course of injections of Prontosil.[19] When Leonard Colebrook learned of the work of Domagk, he decided that he must give Prontosil a trial at Queen Charlotte's.

In fact his first patient was his colleague, Ronald Hare, who was the bacteriologist to the unit. He had pricked his finger on broken glassware, which proved to be contaminated by a culture of streptococci. He developed a severe infection which, spreading up his arm, went on to make him gravely ill with blood poisoning.

Colebrook decided to administer Prontosil by a course of injections. As Hare steadily improved with this treatment (while turning him a bright pink colour), Colebrook's relief was mixed with excitement as he compared this favourable outcome with his wide experience of puerperal fever patients with blood poisoning. Colebrook then went on to treat a series of patients with severe puerperal fever with Prontosil: among 64 mothers there were only three deaths (6.4%) – in contrast to previous experience with a similar group of patients among whom the mortality averaged 25%.[20]

Soon it became clear that Prontosil was broken down in the body to a red dye, and its main constituent the sulphonamide group. Analysis showed that sulphonamides killed streptococci by blocking their nourishment, which allowed the white cells of the blood to engulf the dying bacteria. Chemists used the sulphonamides as the basis for the synthesis of a number of sulpha drugs, which proved valuable in patients with pneumonia and meningitis.

Then, in 1938, Howard Florey, the Professor of Pathology in Oxford, and Ernst Chain, a Jewish refugee from Germany who was a biochemist, began a review of natural anti-bacterial substances. They came across the paper written by Alexander Fleming at St Mary's Hospital in London, in 1929, about his discovery of penicillin. He had picked up a culture dish, already inoculated with staphylococci, on which a stray mould had alighted and grown on the culture medium. As the mould grew its juices had soaked out into the medium, where they had stopped the growth of the staphylococcal colonies, which lay, dead, in a circle around the mould. Fleming had looked further at this mould. He confirmed that the juice from the mould killed micrococci, and because the mould was a specimen of *Penicillium notatum*, he named its active principle 'Penicillin' – it proved to be very unstable if kept for any length of time.[21]

In 1939 Florey, Chain and their colleagues in Oxford decided to look further into the nature of penicillin. Gradually they overcame the difficulties of growing the mould and extracting the active principle from the culture medium on which the mould had grown. Eventually, in May 1940, while the rescue of the British Army from the beaches of Dunkirk was at its height, they had enough penicillin to conduct a crucial experiment to test its potential. They injected eight mice with a lethal dose of streptococci: four were returned to their cage, while the other four received a series of injections of penicillin. They survived, while the untreated four were soon dead. Further experiments confirmed the remarkable properties of penicillin, and the Oxford team embarked on the long process of refining its production, and testing the results. In the process, Florey and Heatley had to go to the USA to secure facilities for the large-scale production of penicillin. As a consequence, penicillin was available in quantity for the treatment of casualties from the invasion of Normandy in June 1944. Detailed trials also began under the Medical Research Council among the civilian population, with very encouraging results. In 1945 the Nobel Prize for Medicine was awarded to Fleming, Florey and Chain.[22]

The Advocates of Cleanliness

It seems strange to us that ordinary notions of hygiene did not lead surgeons to wash their hands and instruments before operating, and to wear a change of clothing, but these instincts were hardly a part of normal life in the early nineteenth century. Water had to be carried, paid for and conserved, and washing of the person and household linen was limited. However, there were signs of change.

James Syme, in the early years of his career, when he worked in the 1830s at Minto House in Edinburgh, was ahead of his time. He 'was most strict in the observance of cleanliness as regards instruments, sponges and hands, especially when recently in contact with any erysipelatous surface or inflammatory discharges',[23] and this always remained his practice.

In the middle of the century he was followed by a select group who believed that surgical help must be offered to the neglected group of women who were literally weighed down by the growth of an ovarian cyst. At a time when any surgery in the abdominal cavity was generally frowned upon, these pioneers gradually developed operative techniques which took particular care over soap and water cleanliness.

The growth of cysts in the ovary is a common problem and, though some are malignant tumours, many are benign. They exert their effects over time through sheer growth in size. In an age when no active treatment was attempted this tendency caused great disability – the stomach was so compressed that little food was taken and the diaphragm was displaced upwards, affecting breathing and the actions of the heart. Some patients presented, wasted and weak, wrapped around an abdominal mass which reached down to their knees. Keith records a patient who needed '4 or 5 gallons of albuminous fluid removed every 3 or 4 weeks'.[24]

Abdominal surgery was virtually unheard of when the first recorded operation to remove an ovarian cyst was performed by Dr Ephraim McDowell in Kentucky in 1809.[25] His patient, Mrs Jane Crawford, had ridden sixty miles on horseback to his surgery,

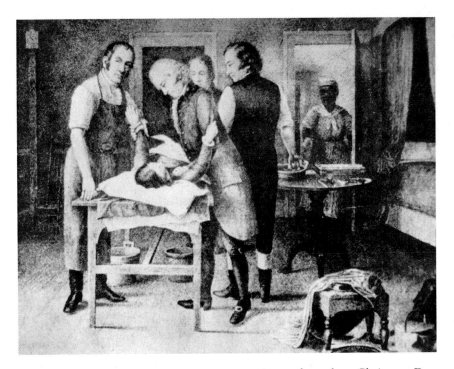

Fig. 3.1. The first recorded ovarian cystectomy, performed on Christmas Day, 1809, by Ephraim McDowell. This drawing was created from memory by a bystander at the operation. (McKay, W.S. *Lawson Tait*, London, 1922)

with her abdominal mass balanced on the horns of the saddle. Persuaded by this resolute patient, McDowell operated in his surgery on Christmas Day, without benefit of general anaesthesia (fig. 3.1). He made a vertical incision nine inches in length, which revealed a tumour too large to be brought out. Fifteen pounds weight of a dirty gelatinous substance were extracted, and this allowed the tumour to be delivered. The narrow stalk, containing the blood supply and fallopian tube, was tied off with strong thread and divided. The tumour, weighing 7½ pounds, was then removed. The intestines were replaced with some difficulty and the long ligature was brought out through the lower end of the incision: this was closed with silk sutures passed through all layers of the abdominal wall. Mrs Crawford had maintained her spirits by repeating the Psalms throughout the procedure: she was up making her own bed on the fifth day. The wound seems to have healed uneventfully and this remarkable lady returned home well after three weeks and lived to the age of 78.

McDowell published an account of this operation, and of three others with recovery, in 1817. As a student he had spent a year in Edinburgh, during 1793–94, and had enjoyed the lectures of Dr John Bell, so he sent a copy of the report to his teacher. However, Bell was ill and in Italy, and his correspondence and practice in Edinburgh were in the hands of John Lizars. In 1824 Lizars gave a full account of McDowell's report.[26] In the following year he removed a large ovarian cyst and the patient survived: this seems to have been the first successful ovariotomy in Britain.

Dr William Jeaffreson of Framlingham in Suffolk was in 1836 the first person to perform an ovariotomy successfully in England, and from 1842 Charles Clay in Manchester performed a series of operations: unfortunately his reports were not precise about his results, and Clay was the subject of much criticism. During the next decade a number of individuals attempted ovariotomy, but there were few successes, and professional opinion on both sides of the Atlantic was that this operation could not be recommended.[27]

It was at this point, in 1857, that Spencer Wells embarked on his pioneer work, which played a large part in the eventual reversal of this opinion. However, at this time, as Wells later remarked, 'ovariotomy was simply nowhere'.[28] Wells, who was the son of a builder in St Albans, qualified MRCS in 1841 and served for some years as a Naval Surgeon. In 1854 he joined the staff of the Samaritan Hospital for Women in London as Dispensary Surgeon. After a year acting as a civilian medical officer in the Crimean War, he returned to begin his particular study of women with ovarian cysts.

Wells made his first report in 1859 when he gave a detailed account of the first five women on whom he had operated. Over time, there were two main reasons for the steady growth of his reputation in this field – one was its volume, with over 1,200 ovariotomies in 25 years, and the other was the consistent honesty and detail of his reports. From the start, every patient and her outcome were declared, with, wherever possible, an autopsy report on any fatal case. Wells's clinical examination of his patients was most careful, and he made few mistakes. He preferred to operate in the patient's home, away from the risks of the hospital; at the Samaritan he isolated the patient with her special nurse and operated in a well-ventilated, bare, cleaned room. At that time he still operated in a frock coat, and only cleaned his instruments after the operation. Marine sponges were used as mops, and were carefully washed out, but they were used from case to case. Wells used a midline incision, and the size of the cyst was reduced by drawing off its fluid content. The stalk was usually crushed in a clamp, the cyst removed, and the clamp on the stalk brought out through the lower end of the incision, where over some days it gradually loosened and came away.[29]

These methods meant that there remained a considerable risk of infection. In 1862 Wells reported on his first fifty patients: a recovery in the case of 33 patients was, in its day, remarkable, but 17 died – one from tetanus, another from a bowel obstruction, and there were a number of cases of 'infection' and 'peritonitis'. 'Exhaustion' was given as a cause of death in other patients, and is a reminder of the extreme weakness of many women by the time they came to operation. It is not surprising that the mortality rate of the first 100 patients was 34%. In 1872, when Wells reported on the fifth set of 100 patients, the mortality rate had fallen to 20%: some deaths were due to infection, but a number continued to be due to Wells's desire to give the benefit of operation to anyone for whom it offered even a slight chance of rescue from a miserable situation.[30]

By 1878 Wells had come, rather slowly, to recognise the value of Lister's work. Before operating he sterilised his instruments in carbolic lotion, rolled up his sleeves and donned a clean gown. He also recognised that he could now safely tie the stalk of the cyst with a sterile silk ligature, and cut this short, before dividing the stalk and removing the cyst. This allowed him to close the whole length of the incision. In 1880 Wells performed his one-thousandth ovariotomy, and in the last 112 patients the mortality rate was down to 10.6%.[31] The *British Medical Journal* commented that he 'had rescued the operation from the discredit into which it had fallen and established it, in the opinion of the profession here and abroad, as a thoroughly legitimate and marvellously successful surgical operation'.[32]

A friend and contemporary of Wells was Thomas Keith who is, in comparison, little known, but who had an equally remarkable career. Born in 1827, Keith came from St Cyrus in Kincardineshire, attended Aberdeen Grammar School, and went on to study medicine in Edinburgh. He was apprenticed in 1845 to Professor J. Y. Simpson, with whom his brother George already worked, so Thomas was most probably present on the evening in November 1847 when chloroform received its first test. Keith graduated MD in 1848 and served as house surgeon to James Syme for fifteen months. (In later years Keith warmly acknowledged his debt to Syme, who taught him the surgical principles of simplicity, painstaking technique and absolute cleanliness.) In 1852 Keith joined his brother George in his busy general practice, and for twenty years he was his partner, but Keith had always entertained the hope of becoming a surgeon, and an unusual story is told of how he became an ovariotomist.[33]

In 1862 a workman was repairing windows in Keith's house, and he mentioned to Keith that his wife suffered from an abdominal tumour. After several requests Keith agreed to see her, and he found the signs of an ovarian cyst. Keith had to tell the couple that operation for this condition was not accepted by most doctors, often proved fatal, and that he had no experience of such an operation. However, both partners were desperate and continued to press Keith to operate. At this time he held no hospital appointment, and he knew of no surgeon who would undertake such a case. The couple persisted and after much thought Keith determined to go ahead. He cleared and cleaned a room in the couple's dwelling, and before the operation the husband spent the night building up a large stock of boiled water. 'In this his first case Keith laid the foundations of his success – chemical cleanliness is what he aimed at ... cleanliness of the patient and of everything that was to come in contact with her.'[34]

Keith's emotions as he prepared to open the abdomen of his patient in September 1862 must have been profound, for he knew that if he failed there were many colleagues who would accuse him of malpractice. He went ahead and exposed a semi-solid cyst which proved to weigh 25 pounds (11.4 kilos). After a clamp was placed across the stalk it was divided, and the cyst was removed: the clamp was then placed on the abdominal wall and the incision closed around it, where it gradually loosened. The patient recovered, as did Keith's second patient from whom, after dividing 'firm and extensive parietal, omental and intestinal adhesions', he removed a cyst weighing 45 pounds (20 kilos).[35] (In retrospect it is extraordinary to think of Keith performing these two operations, without previous experience, and dealing more or less unaided with many difficult adhesions, which are still a problem for modern surgeons.)

Encouraged by these results, early in 1863 Keith set about converting the loft of his house in Great Stuart Street, in Edinburgh's New Town, into an operating theatre which was reserved for ovarian operations.

The third patient, aged only 24 and 'in the last stage of disease', proved also to be of great technical difficulty. The cyst was large (63 pounds, 29.5 kilos), 'adhesions very firm and extensive ... at least 20 vessels tied'.[36] Keith found his patient dead in her bed next morning, with her night nurse, dead drunk, lying on the floor beside the patient.[37] This would have been one of the cases on whom 'I operated against my own judgement, and at the entreaty of women whose lives had become intolerable ... In five I would have been only too glad to have declined interference, but did not feel warranted in withholding a probable chance of life, however small.' Keith sought the opinion of colleagues in these cases before consenting to operate, but it required real courage to proceed when medical opinion was still against the operation and he himself was relatively inexperienced. In only his fourth patient, in March 1863, Keith was presented with the largest tumour he ever removed: remarkably he undertook this in a cottage in the country. The tumour lay not only over the thighs but on the legs, and after removal weighed 'upwards of 120 pounds (55 kilos)'. Keith noted that 'its removal was the most formidable proceeding I was ever concerned in'.[38] 'When the patient was put to bed, apparently moribund, Dr Keith said to the nurse that she would not give her much trouble as she would soon die: some weeks later the woman had the pleasure of telling Dr Keith what she had heard him say.'[39]

Keith was a good friend of Spencer Wells, and he shared with him a dedication to accurate surgical audit. Every patient was recorded, with comments and final outcome. In his first year, 1862–63, Keith operated on nine patients, the youngest 16 and the oldest 52 years of age, with six recoveries. In 1864, 16 patients came to operation, with four deaths, so in the first 25 women the mortality rate was 28%: nine had tumours weighing over 20 kilograms, with extensive adhesions to the intestines, so this is a very low figure when set against the rarity of abdominal surgery at the time.[40]

A later tribute to Keith recalls 'a weird-looking, gaunt, silent man, blessed with a passionate desire to succour his kind, gifted with an absolute indifference to accepted opinion. He would have nursed and fed his case with his own hands, and nearly broke his heart when all was in vain. With no hospital appointment at his back; with the countenance of a very small minority of the profession; at his own expense and risk; sustained by his own personal devotion – he operated on one poor woman after another, learning from his difficulties, and still diminishing his mortality'[41] (fig. 3.2).

In January 1867 Keith wrote a detailed report on each of his 51 treated patients, and he could say that 'of the 40 patients saved by ovariotomy, all are now alive and well'.[42] He gave details of twelve patients on whom, for very good reasons, he had declined

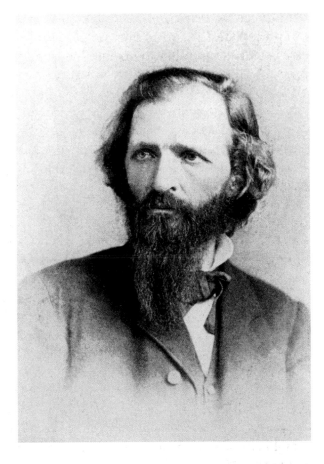

Fig. 3.2.
Thomas Keith,
1827–95, the
Edinburgh general
practitioner
who carried
out 300 ovarian
cystectomies.
(Skene, 'Thomas
Keith', *Brooklyn
Medical Journal,*
1896)

to operate. In 1870 Keith gave a report on a further fifty patients.[43] Overall there were 19 deaths – 11 in the first and eight in the second series – of which four were due to malignant disease, one to the complications of chloroform anaesthesia and eight to sepsis. This record can be compared with the figure of 23 deaths in the third group of 100 patients published by Spencer Wells in 1869.[44] Both Wells and Keith reached the conclusion in the same year – 1867 – that chloroform was not a wholly safe anaesthetic. Keith already had his doubts, and in January 1867 a patient died on the sixth day from its toxic effects. Both men thereafter used ether and were among the first to recognise that, although in expert hands it had good results, chloroform was not proving to be a safe anaesthetic for general use.

During 1867 Lister published his first two papers on the antiseptic principle. Mindful of the trouble he had experienced with post-operative sepsis, in spite of his meticulous care, Keith was among the first to visit Lister in Glasgow. There he saw the effect which carbolic acid lotion had on dirty compound fractures. From that time Keith used antiseptics in various ways before, in 1876, adopting the full Listerian method. This entailed using the carbolic acid spray set 8 feet away from the operation site, bathing it in a fine mist. Instruments were soaked in 1-in-20 carbolic lotion, and hands and linen thoroughly washed and rinsed in the lotion.[45] Dr Marion Sims, the famous American gynaecologist, came to watch Keith operate and commented: 'Keith never hurries, he does nothing for display, but I have never seen anyone cut down to the peritoneal cavity more quickly, though cautiously, remove a tumour with greater celerity, or close up the external wound more rapidly – the time that he dallies is when he comes to arrest any haemorrhage – he leaves no bleeding points, never closes the wound until all oozing has ceased, until he has tied perhaps 20 points with fine catgut.'[46]

In the following year a leader in *The Scotsman* of 20 November 1879 saluted 'a great deed in surgery', with the completion by Keith of 300 ovariotomies: only three women had died in the final group of 100 patients.[47]

The select group of surgeons who espoused cleanliness was completed by Lawson Tait, who graduated in Edinburgh in 1866, by which time both Wells and Keith were experienced ovariotomists. In 1871 he joined the staff of the Women's Hospital in Birmingham. He never subscribed to the germ theory of surgical sepsis: he depended on thorough washing of hands and instruments with soap and water, but he took great care with his sponges, which he used to mop out the wound, and after thorough washing he soaked them in carbolic lotion for a week. He used silk ligatures sterilised in boiling water.[48] This combination of antiseptic and aseptic methods helped Tait to accomplish 136 ovariotomies during 1886 without a death.[49]

In 1878, ten years after he had adopted antiseptic principles, Keith reported on his experience:

Antiseptics are a great comfort and relief to the operator, and ovariotomy is not the operation it was ... no one knows but who has experienced it the anxiety and weariness of spirit with which the struggle against the blood poison was carried on. The worry to get chemical cleanness in one's hands, in the surroundings of the patient, has passed away. Now there is a feeling of confidence and security. With an 1 in 20 carbolic solution and a nail brush I am safe ... this long despised operation is now the safest of all the great surgical operations, at least judging from these results – 3 deaths in the last 75 operations. Whatever may appear in the future of antiseptics in surgery, the name of Joseph Lister, who put us on the right way, will not be forgotten.[50]

These developments extended over a period of some 70 years. At its end, in 1860, Professor Lister was embarking on his nine pivotal years in Glasgow which would see him take the vital first steps in what became his life's work.

Professor Lister in Glasgow

In the early autumn of 1861 Professor Lister was able, after 18 months of delays, to embark on the full range of his duties. Not the least of these was the requirement to deliver personally a series of 92 lectures on the Principles of Surgery. These took place at 8.30 a.m. on five days in the week, and must have placed substantial demands on the stamina of his students as well as Lister himself. He would leave 17 Woodside Place, enter his brougham, and drive the 2½ miles through the thronged streets of the city to the University. One of his students has described how Lister used 'deliberate and clear language, without show or ornament, but rendered piquant by a slight stammer, and an occasional flash of quiet humour'.[51] Lister himself tells how the size and enthusiasm of the class was enough 'to cause both ideas and language to flow in a manner that really surprises me'.[52] It cannot have been easy for a lecturer to hold the attention of a large and lively class at that early hour, but Lister's assets were his natural modesty, combined with his enthusiasm for science and for surgery.

The first 44 lectures were devoted to Inflammation, and here
Lister already had the background of the hours of observation
which he and Agnes had spent over two years, studying the
changes in the frog's foot. It must have been refreshing to
listen to someone telling of his original observations rather than
receiving textbook teaching. Throughout his life Lister never lost
the earnestness of his Quaker ancestry, but this was linked with
the sheer enthusiasm he felt for his subject, and for the sense
of privilege which he – and in turn his students – enjoyed in
possessing, or acquiring, the knowledge which enabled them to
provide good care for their patients.

This broad subject of Inflammation covered a large proportion
of the problems encountered by the Victorian surgeon. Every day
he would see acute inflammation, manifest as boils, carbuncles,
erysipelas and cellulitis, and often encounter the serious childhood
complaint of acute osteomyelitis. These acute infections were
particularly common in a population living and working in
crowded and dangerous situations, and in those days (some eighty
years before the arrival of any specific treatment in the form of
the sulphonamides and then the antibiotics) they could progress
to a fatal septicaemia.

Lister then had to deal with the equally common group
of Chronic Inflammatory Diseases – syphilis with its many
manifestations, and tuberculous disease – both directly associated
with the prevailing social conditions. At this time – the early
1860s – there was no recognition of the cause of these diseases
by infection with specific germs. Tuberculosis was known by
various names such as struma, scrofula, caries, and it was generally
considered to be a hereditary condition. This was understandable
at a time when the Scottish Census of 1871 showed that 'in the
City of Glasgow 41 out of every 100 families lived in houses
having only one room',[53] which provided ideal circumstances for
cross-infection. Another twenty years would pass before Robert
Koch in Berlin would demonstrate the bacterial basis for the
human and bovine forms of tuberculosis, but it had for long been
clear that this disease had many varieties. The lungs (phthisis),
the spine (Pott's disease), bones and joints of the limbs (caries),
lymph glands in the neck (scrofula), and the abdomen, intestines

and the urinary tract were all affected. Only years later would it become clear that milk from infected cows was largely responsible for many of these manifestations of tuberculosis, especially in children (p. 169).

Cumulatively, tuberculosis would continue to place a great workload on the hospital services of the country, and orthopaedic hospitals and sanatoria were established to provide long-term in-patient treatment: a demand which would only ease as specific antibiotic treatment became a reality in the mid-1940s. Among other subjects, Lister spoke of the knock-knees and bowed legs which were then very common among the slum children: we now know that these were due to their poor diet and few chances of playing in the sun, which meant that they grew up deficient in vitamin D, and suffering from rickets.

Further lectures were devoted to the wide range of accidents which the students would have to manage, arising in the busy streets, mines, factories, shipyards and the many crowded homes.

There was barely a mention of abdominal surgery because in those days the peritoneal cavity was hardly ever opened by the general surgeon. This subject was already being explored by the few pioneers who were devoting their skills to the removal of large ovarian cysts, but generally this was considered to be too dangerous an undertaking.

The lecture over, Lister and his students would make the short journey up the High Street to the Royal Infirmary, which lay beside Glasgow Cathedral. The main building was designed by Robert Adam and had opened in 1794. Behind this lay the Fever Hospital which had been opened in 1829: this allowed for the separation of patients with typhus and typhoid fever. On the third side of the square a new Surgical Hospital had just been built, and it opened in May 1861. There were eight wards, each holding sixteen beds, and at the top of the building, under the dome, lay the operating theatre which had seating for 200 students (fig. 3.3).

Lister had charge of two main wards – the male accident ward on the ground floor and his female ward on the first floor – and he must have had high hopes as he entered on his work. There

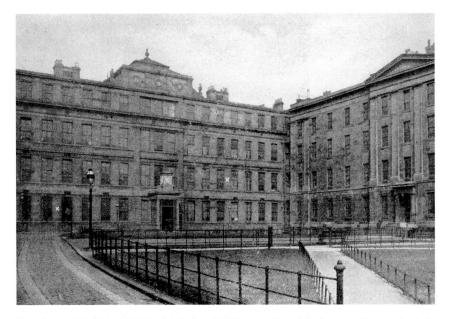

Fig. 3.3. The Surgical Block of the old Glasgow Royal Infirmary lies to the left. It was opened in May 1861, five months before Lister started to work in it. His male accident ward, No 24, was on the ground floor, to the left of the entrance, which lay under the clock. His female ward was on the first floor, to the right of the entrance. The surgical amphitheatre lay beneath the dome. The Fever Block, opened in 1829, lies on the right: Macewen's wards were on the top floor, close to the right angle between the two blocks. (Cameron, *Reminiscences*)

were some 2,500–3,000 surgical admissions to the Infirmary each year, of which about one-quarter were due to accidental injury. Yet the number of operations performed was remarkably low – in 1861, the year of Lister's arrival, 212 operations were carried out, about four in each week. Of these, 83 were amputations, of which 29 (35%) were fatal.[54] It was not until November of 1861 that Lister performed his first operation, and this must have been quite a test, performed in front of staff and students who would be ready enough to note any mistakes. However, Lister was able to report to his mother: 'I had not hoped to be able so entirely to disregard the throng of spectators ... it was curious how entirely absent any shade of anxiety was during the whole proceedings.'[55]

In 1861 surgery was at something of a standstill. The advantages of the ready availability of anaesthesia were fully utilised, but this had not led to any significant extension of the range of surgery. One great inhibition hung over the work of surgeons, and this was well expressed by Lister as he surveyed his work in the new building – 'to the disappointment of all this noble structure proved extremely unhealthy. Pyaemia, erysipelas and hospital gangrene soon showed themselves, and my patients suffered from these evils in a way which was sickening and heartrending'.[56] His house surgeon later recalled that 'more than once as he entered his carriage after visiting the wards, I have seen Lister deeply distressed and agitated'.[57] This was a general experience – von Volkmann, Professor of Surgery in Halle, and Lister's contemporary, was faced with so much sepsis that he seriously considered closing the hospital. Many surgeons took 'the fatalistic view that septic diseases of wounds were unavoidable accidents, as much acts of God as hail in harvest, and matters therefore for which the surgeon had no personal responsibility'.[58] For some, sepsis was not a major concern, and the story is told that Sir Astley Cooper – one of the most skilful surgeons of his time – was asked to remove a sebaceous cyst from the scalp of King William IV. On the day after the operation the King greeted Cooper quite coolly. Later, Cooper asked the King's Physician the reason for this and was told: 'I would have put on a clean shirt, or at least have washed my hands, before I waited on His Majesty'. Cooper looked at his blood-spattered shirt and hands and replied, 'God bless me, so I ought – and the King is so very particular.'[59] The general opinion was that sepsis was due to overcrowding, dirt and 'bad air', and the design of the new Surgical Hospital reflected these beliefs with its lofty wards, many windows and well-spaced beds.

The arrival of Lister in Glasgow coincided with a time of great activity in the city. The many cotton mills of the early nineteenth century were giving way to tremendous developments in engineering, based on the rich deposits of coal and ore in the region. Soon the Clyde shipyards were producing two-thirds of British tonnage, and the railway workshops were supplying the world with steam engines, rolling stock and track. Working conditions were often unsafe and the narrow streets were thronged with traffic, so accidents were frequent. Labour was flowing into the city from the surrounding countryside, greatly supplemented by the consequences of the Irish potato famine and the Highland Clearances. Many of these immigrants were destitute, and consequently gathered in the closes of the High Street and Gallowgate, where 'they were accommodated cheaply through existing buildings being subdivided and their backcourts filled in with additional buildings. Housing conditions in such areas were appalling simply because so many had no alternative but to accept them'[60] (fig. 3.4). Speaking some years later, Dr J. B. Russell, the Medical Officer of Health (who had been a member of Lister's first class in Glasgow), said:

> But what does that mean? It means that 126,000 people *live* in those one-roomed, and 228,000 in those two-roomed, houses ... I ask you to imagine yourselves with your appetites and passions, your bodily necessities and functions, your sense of propriety, your births, your sicknesses, your deaths, your children – in short, your *lives* in the whole round of the seen and the unseen, suddenly shrivelled and shrunk into such conditions of space. There [the children] die and their little bodies are placed on a table or a dresser, so as to be somewhat out of the way of their brothers and sisters who play and sleep and eat in their ghastly company ... their exhausted air and poor and perverse feeding fill our streets with bandy-legged children.[61]

These social conditions can never have been far away from the medical staff and students in Glasgow in the middle of the nineteenth century, as each day they were confronted with such sights, sounds and smells as they walked and drove up the High Street to the University and the Infirmary. It was the sufferers from these conditions who were their patients. Admission to the Infirmary was more or less limited to those who could not afford to pay a doctor. The contamination of wounds with the dirt of factories and streets, and the clothes of patients who could rarely wash them or themselves, produced conditions in the wards in which blankets and mattresses soon, in turn, became contaminated. At that time, with no clear idea of the source of wound infection or its prevention, it is not surprising that

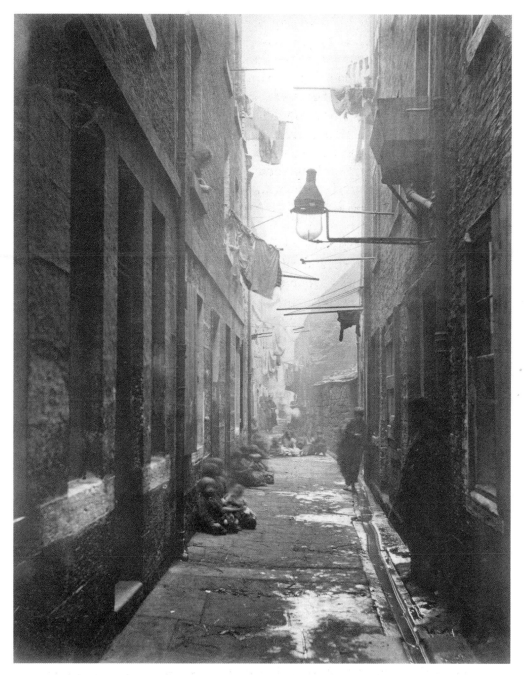

Fig. 3.4. Alleyway off the High Street of Glasgow, photographed by Thomas Annan in the 1860s. These tenements are typical of the slum property surrounding the old University buildings on the High Street. (Mitchell Library, Glasgow)

the accident wards of the new hospital 'proved to be extremely unhealthy'.[62] Hector Cameron, who became Lister's house surgeon in 1867, remembered later that, as a student, 'I myself have seen as many as five men die from pyaemia following amputation of a limb for injury in one week, while others lay ill with pyaemia and hospital gangrene'.[63]

However, it is a mistake to imagine that elective surgery was not practised. When pain or deformity made life more or less unbearable, then operation was offered to the patient, and if consent was given it was performed – with misgivings on both sides, but with the hope that it would go on to satisfactory healing. This was the background to a series of operations reported by Lister in 1865 – in fact the last occasion on which he wrote a detailed paper devoted solely to surgical anatomy and technique.

During 1862 Lister became interested in tuberculous disease (caries) in the bones of the wrist, which most often affected young people, and presented the surgeon with a real problem. All too often this had been treated by amputation, yet as Lister himself said: 'to save a human hand from amputation, and to restore its usefulness, is an object well worthy of any labour involved in it'.[64] He had seen the good results which Professor Syme obtained by treating tuberculosis at the elbow by excision of the joint, which had often resulted in a useful limb, but at the wrist the record of joint excision was not encouraging. Lister's careful study of this subject reveals several characteristics of his approach to surgery and to his patients.

During 1862 Lister had cared for a 17-year-old miner who had fallen fifty feet down a mineshaft. He sustained a fracture of the thigh and a compound dislocation of the left wrist, with the lower end of the radius and ulna protruding from the wound, and severe disturbance of the tendons to the wrist and fingers. Lister removed the exposed bone, cleaned the wound and splinted the arm. He commenced early passive and active movements of the wrist, and was pleasantly surprised to find, after five months, that the patient had a hand 'nearly as supple and strong as the other'.

This experience led Lister to hope that excision of the wrist for tuberculosis was worth pursuing, and his account of his experience occupies 10 pages of three issues of *The Lancet* during March

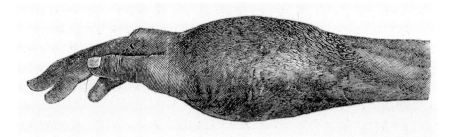

Fig. 3.5. A case of tuberculosis of the wrist joint. (Lister, 'On excision of the wrist for caries')

and April of 1865 (fig. 3.5).[65] He had learned from tuberculosis at the elbow that the whole of the cartilage lining the joint had to be removed to ensure complete excision of the affected tissue. At the wrist this would mean quite a wide removal of the bone and cartilage lining the joint, so the outcome would remain in some doubt. The first patient in this trial was a woman of 40, a millworker, admitted in October 1862, with active disease in the right wrist, which at first was treated with splintage. This was unavailing, with the patient continuing to suffer severe pain, so in April 1863 Lister operated. He excised diseased bone at the lower ends of the radius and ulna, the small carpal bones of the wrist, and the inner ends of the metacarpal bones, measuring overall some 5 cm. The wound healed well and movements began, but then the woman suddenly left the hospital and was not seen for five months. On re-examination the operation site was well healed but very stiff: manipulation restored some movement and when last seen two years after the operation she had a strong mobile wrist.

Encouraged by this belated but promising result, Lister went on to treat his second patient, Margaret, aged 14 years, a sewing-machine operator, who had had a swollen painful right wrist for five months. Several abscesses required drainage, and these left unhealed discharging wounds. Quite a wide excision of all the carpal bones and the adjacent radius and ulna was required, but the wounds healed well, and movements were started early. Three months later she could pick up a bandage and at six months

Margaret was knitting stockings. At this time a nurse on the ward taught her to write (there being no compulsory schooling at this time). After a further six months Lister received a letter from Margaret, 'well written with the affected hand, asking for a certificate of sound healing for her employer. Eighteen months after the operation Margaret reported that she was earning 10 shillings a week, and had been told she was one of the firm's best hands.[66]

After describing six patients in detail, Lister gives a full description of his technique, and the long period of after-care. In the third paper he describes four more patients, in three of whom the occurrence of hospital gangrene after the operation required vigorous treatment. In all he treated 15 patients, two were as young as 9 and 12 years old, seven were in their teens and four in their early twenties; only two were over 40 years of age. The final result in 10 patients was restoration of normal function, with another two progressing well, while in one the prognosis was uncertain. All these arms were, of necessity, shorter because some 5–7 cm of bone had been excised, but the space left had to some extent filled in with bony tissue. It may seem remarkable that so much recovery of function can occur after the removal of so much bone, but with close supervision over many months, and plenty of what is now called physiotherapy, this was achieved. Two patients died. One already had advanced pulmonary tuberculosis, but operation was undertaken to relieve intense pain at the wrist, and this yielded seven weeks of 'freedom from his previous suffering' before death occurred. In the other patient, a youth of 21, also with tuberculosis of the lungs, post-operative wound infection spread into and up the veins to the elbow: the next day a spreading bloodstream infection was confirmed when he had a severe rigor. Lister thought the pyaemia might be arrested if he performed an amputation at the shoulder but this proved ineffective, and the patient died with lung complications. This patient, and the others whose recovery was complicated by hospital gangrene in the wound, are a reminder of the risks involved in even the most careful elective surgery in the days before the development of the antiseptic principle.[67]

Lister's long, detailed paper gives a foretaste of all the papers which he wrote as he worked out this principle over the years

– there was complete candour over the details of technique and outcome in each patient, with the inclusion of a number of personal touches about the lives of his patients. He displayed an interest in them which was unusual for his time, illustrated by his rule that he always accompanied the anaesthetised patient from the theatre to the ward, taking control of the head – an important point when patients had to be carried up and down stairs on a blanket. Lister was well known for performing his own post-operative dressings (and for the consequent length of his ward rounds), but this meant that he truly knew the results of his work.

'Excision of the wrist for caries' was published early in 1865, just at the time when the trial of the carbolic acid treatment of compound fractures was getting under way. Although at first unremarked, the results of that trial and their subsequent development were to become Lister's major preoccupation for the remainder of his life.

These had been full years for Lister who, in addition to his hospital work, 'had pretty frequent calls from private practice'. He was Secretary to the Medical Faculty, which entailed considerable correspondence, all in longhand.[68] At home, Joseph and Agnes were often at work in the laboratory, at that time engaged on his studies of the mechanisms which prevent and promote clotting of the blood. These were presented as the Croonian Lecture to the Royal Society of London in June 1863. In 1861 the Listers were visited by Joseph's father and mother, who travelled from London in a saloon carriage of the Great Northern Railway. Isabella found the journey very fatiguing, but she soon recovered in the Lister's 'excellent house at the West End, airy, with a space of lawn and trees in front'.[69] In 1862 James Syme came over to attend the launch into the Clyde of *The Black Prince*, only the second British ironclad warship to be built. During 1860–63 the Listers housed their nephew, Marcus Beck, during the time that he was a medical student in Glasgow. On Sunday afternoons Joseph and Marcus would often take a walk together, and on one excursion to Loch Lomond they decided to climb Ben Lomond: the day was warm and they soon discarded their waistcoats, took a drink of milk at a cottage and at the top admired a view which Marcus described as 'most glorious'.[70]

The marriage of Joseph and Agnes was, in those days, unusual, for they were real partners, with Agnes bringing a keen intelligence to bear as his assistant, amanuensis and real collaborator in his experiments. This extended to his work, where her letters expressed her keen concerns over Joseph's first lectures and operations, as well as his pioneering investigations on his patients. It seems certain that their progress must often have been discussed, and one imagines many a worried morning when Lister left for the Infimary after strong encouragement.

In 1864 there was an interruption for some months when Agnes went down to Upton to care for Isabella who was seriously ill with erysipelas, and she finally died in September of that year. This left Joseph Jackson alone, and the considerable correspondence which he had conducted with Joseph over the years became all the more important to J.J. This had always been a free and frequent exchange, with Joseph placing great reliance on his father's mature advice.

CHAPTER FOUR

The Birth of the Antiseptic Principle, 1865–1870

Lister's Eleven Patients

The occasion which saw the origin of the antiseptic system is well recorded. It was a winter afternoon in late 1864 when Professor Lister, in the company of Dr Thomas Anderson, the Professor of Chemistry, set out from the University of Glasgow to walk home through the busy streets. They were discussing the subject of putrefaction, a condition which can affect any organic substance left exposed to the atmospheric air, whether it be a jug of milk or an open wound.

During that walk Professor Anderson drew Lister's attention to some recent papers by Louis Pasteur, the French biologist; these had been published in the French scientific press, which Lister did not usually see. He speedily obtained these journals and soon recognised the kernel of Pasteur's observations: he had shown that 'the septic property of the atmosphere depended not on the oxygen or any gaseous constituent, but on minute organisms suspended in it, which owed their origin to their vitality'.[1]

It was Lister's habit to apply 'acute reasoning to the interpretation of the results of accurate observation and experiment'.[2] This allowed him to progress to the idea that 'decomposition in an open injured part might be avoided – without excluding the air – by applying as a dressing some material capable of destroying the life of the floating particles'.[3] To illustrate the truth of this germ theory of putrefaction Lister performed an experiment based on the work of Pasteur.

I introduced portions of the same specimen of urine into four glass flasks, each about one-third full. After washing their necks, I drew them out with a spirit lamp into tubes about one line [2 mm] in diameter, and then bent three of them at various acute angles, while the fourth was left short and vertical, though equally narrow (fig. 4.1). Each was then boiled

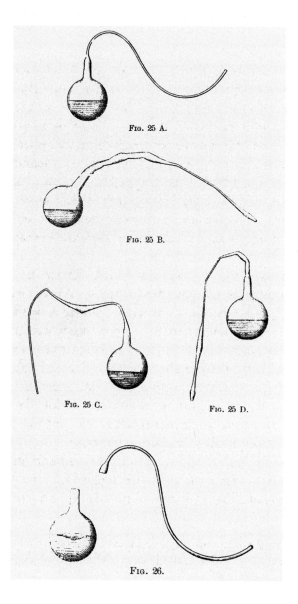

FIG. 25 A.

FIG. 25 B.

FIG. 25 C.   FIG. 25 D.

FIG. 26.

Fig. 4.1. Pasteur's Flasks. At first all five flasks were identical, with wide straight necks, and all filled with fresh broth. After washing the necks, four flasks had their necks heated and drawn out into thin, angular shapes. The neck of the fifth flask was left straight and open. Lister conducted a similar experiment, with results recorded here. (Pasteur, L., *Oeuvres de Pasteur*, Paris, 1922. Tome II, 260–1)

for 5 minutes to kill organisms, steam issuing freely from the orifice, after which they were left, the ends of the necks all open, so that air could pass in and out freely, in obedience to the condensation and expansion caused by the diurnal changes of temperature The bending of the necks in 3 of the flasks was with the view of intercepting particles of dust which, according to the germ theory, are the cause of putrefaction. The fourth neck was left short and vertical, to afford opportunity for dust to fall into the liquid.[4]

The flasks were left undisturbed, allowing air to pass freely out and in along the four tubes. At the end of three months the urine was still clear in the three flasks with bent tubing, while 'in the vessel with the short upright neck two different kinds of fungi appeared and grew steadily'.[5] All four flasks would have had equal quantities of air moved in and out, but in those with convoluted tubing the dust in the air must have been trapped, and prevented from reaching the urine. By the time Lister wrote this account the urine in the three flasks had remained perfectly clear for some years, although all four flasks had been regularly moved to show to successive classes.

On his teaching rounds in the accident wards Lister had often spoken to his students about 'the frequency of disastrous infective consequences in compound fractures, contrasted with the complete immunity from danger to life and limb in simple fractures', in which skin was unbroken. Lister realised that he now had an explanation for this difference: the three flasks with their convoluted necks were reproducing the action of the skin, keeping dust and its germs away from a surface open to putrefaction. He realised that he had in his wards patients on whom he could test out 'a material capable of destroying floating particles'.[6]

In the course of 1864 Lister had read of 'the remarkable effects produced by carbolic acid* upon the sewage of the town of Carlisle'; these included 'the prevention of odour and the

---

* Creosote, which is derived from coal tar, is a crude form of carbolic acid. When it is distilled creosote yields carbolic acid (phenol) of varying degrees of purity.

destruction of entozoa, which usually infest cattle fed upon the sewage which farmers spread on their fields'.[7] Lister theorised that if carbolic acid could destroy entozoa it should disinfect the contaminated tissues of a compound fracture brought in from the streets. He decided to try the effect of painting these exposed tissues with swabs soaked in carbolic acid. In early trials he noted that the acid also had the useful effect of lessening the pain of such a wound, and that it formed a clot, when mixed with blood, which acted as a form of antiseptic dressing. After two false starts in early 1865, Lister developed a promising method of treatment, and gradually he accumulated a series of cases. He was literally feeling his way, studying each successive patient and modifying his methods accordingly. Lister kept careful notes on each of the patients he treated with antiseptics, and a full account is contained in his first report on the treatment of compound fractures.[8]

The first patient, a boy of 11, had been run over by the wheel of a cart in August 1865, causing a fracture of the mid-shaft of the left tibia, with an open wound in the overlying skin, 1½ inches (4 cm) long. This was thoroughly cleaned, covered with lint soaked in carbolic acid, and the limb splinted. The lad did well, the fracture uniting in six weeks. Lister commented that the open wound was small, though close to the fracture, and he felt that the case 'might have done well under ordinary treatment'.

The second patient was a labourer who, in September 1865, sustained a kick from a horse which fractured his right tibia: the skin wound was bleeding freely. The limb was dressed and splinted as in the first case and at the end of two weeks the wound was clean and all but healed. Lister had to leave Glasgow at this point and he was 'deeply mortified' to learn on his return that this small unhealed wound had been attacked by hospital gangrene, and the leg had been amputated. (This was a striking comment on the risks to which anyone with an open wound, lying in those days in a busy ward, was liable.)

After these two inconclusive cases, Lister knew that the carbolic acid regime needed a sterner test, and he had to wait for eight months until, in May 1866, his third patient was admitted – a youth of 21 whose left leg had been struck by a heavy iron box which fell from a crane. Both the tibia and fibula were broken and there was severe injury to the skin and tissues at the level of the fractures. The limb was swollen with blood and this was squeezed out, the wound freely treated with swabs soaked in carbolic acid, and the leg splinted. Lister wrote that 'on the fourth day – the critical period with reference to suppuration – the limb was free from pain, the calf less tense, and the patient had enjoyed his food after a good night's rest'. He made a smooth recovery, and after six months was walking normally on a strong leg.

In the following month James, aged 10, had his right arm caught between a revolving belt and a shaft driven by a steam engine. Two minutes elapsed before the power could be cut off and the movement of the belting stopped: consequently the arm was badly mauled and both radius and ulna were broken. The upper end of the ulna was protruding through an extensive skin wound. Lister sawed off the exposed shaft of the ulna, excised lacerated muscle, and then applied 'carbolic acid freely to the whole interior of the wound, including the exposed bone'. The limb was dressed and splinted, as was a closed fracture of the lower right humerus. Next day the lad had a good appetite and had slept well. He slowly recovered, with 'a very useful hand'.[9]

These were two more serious injuries, and the period of waiting whilst they slowly progressed must have been a time of considerable anxiety for Lister. At this time the accepted treatment for compound fractures of this severity was immediate amputation, to forestall the almost inevitable severe infection which would have developed in the open wound. Lister was well aware that there were colleagues who would not be slow to criticise if this experimental treatment had failed. At the same time, he would have had a growing hope that these favourable results would indicate that he was working on a sound principle. His next patient, admitted a fortnight later, caused particular anxiety.

On 23 June 1866 Charles, 'a fine intelligent boy', aged 7, was knocked down by a crowded omnibus, one wheel going over his right leg. The whole of the inner side of the leg was laid open, exposing a fractured tibia, and there was another wound over the broken fibula: the lad was in severe haemorrhagic shock. Lister thought seriously about immediate amputation, but doubted whether Charles could stand the additional shock of such an operation, He could feel a pulse on the front of the foot, and this led him to believe that the leg could survive, and that he should use the antiseptic treatment. Under chloroform, Lister 'applied carbolic acid with great freedom, the contused mass being repeatedly squeezed, to induce the liquid to insinuate itself into all the interstices', including the fracture sites. The flayed skin of the leg was then replaced, the wound packed with carbolic dressings, and a plaster board splint applied. After an anxious five days the pulse steadied, appetite returned and the boy was sleeping well. The main wound, some 8 inches (20 cm) long and 6 inches (15 cm) wide, was clean, and healing at its margins, by the end of the second week. Then, during the third week, hospital gangrene attacked the wound over the fibula, and required very active treatment. Under chloroform, Lister scraped away all the grey sloughs, and cleaned the whole area with strong nitric acid. In the main wound the lower end of the tibia lay bare and white, and Lister feared that it might well be dead: amputation was again considered. However, as the days went by the healing wound showed that the tibia had acquired a pink hue, and new tissue was extending over the surface of both ends of the tibia. Signs of hospital gangrene then returned, and as a last resort Charles was moved to an airy room in another part of the hospital, and from then on healing continued. By January 1867 the wounds were healed, the fracture site was firm, and the patient was allowed up, to bear weight. He finally left hospital in March of that year, nine months after the injury. Lister's account of this patient covers two closely printed pages of *The Lancet*. and was typical of the close day-to-day care which always marked his practice.[10]

These three patients had provided a severe testing of the antiseptic system, and the final successful outcome could have given real support to Lister's growing belief that the scientific basis of his experiment was sound. Over the next six months five more patients were treated for a severe compound fracture – four involved the femur or tibia, one the radius and ulna of a woman who had fallen downstairs. Several of these patients were admitted to the beds of other wards which happened to be on duty, and now that Lister's methods were well known they had been treated by their house-surgeons, with the agreement of Lister's colleagues.

All five experienced sound healing of the fracture, but there was a late death.

This patient, a quarry worker, was buried under a heavy fall of rocks and sustained a compound fracture of the right thigh. He was carried on a litter to Helensburgh, and thence travelled by train into Glasgow, arriving at the Infirmary some six hours after injury. His progress was probably slowed by the delay before the contaminated wound could be treated, but finally the fracture united, and the knee was mobilised, although there was still an unhealed wound. At this point, fourteen weeks after the injury, this wound began to bleed and, in spite of ligature of the popliteal artery, behind the knee joint, the patient soon developed a fatal torrential haemorrhage. The autopsy showed that a loose, needle-shaped spicule of bone had penetrated the popliteal artery – a sad ending due to a mechanical complication of the fracture, rather than a failure of the antiseptic system.[11]

Eight of Lister's ten patients, with injuries of varying degrees of complexity, had left hospital with a soundly healed limb. There was one amputation, performed in Lister's absence, and the late death just described. At that time, and in other hands, we can be reasonably sure that more than half of these eight patients would have had an immediate amputation. It should also be remembered that this trial had been conducted in very unfavourable conditions, with Lister's accident wards in early 1865 'among the unhealthiest in the whole surgical division of the Glasgow Royal Infirmary'.[12] The wards were constantly full, the nursing staff had little training, bed linen was not regularly changed, and many wounds were septic, with free discharge of pus. Most patients were poorly nourished, they had few facilities for washing, and most had been injured in streets and factories which were rarely cleaned. This was, in fact, a remarkable, though restricted, series, which had been tentatively embarked upon, but brought to an impressive conclusion. Lister modestly wrote: 'I have had some rather sorrowful experiences in bringing the method of treatment to a trustworthy state, but this I now think I have most satisfactorily done'[13] (fig. 4.2).

Lister did not find it easy to write, but when he did take up his pen (in many cases it was Agnes who was the scribe) he entered into

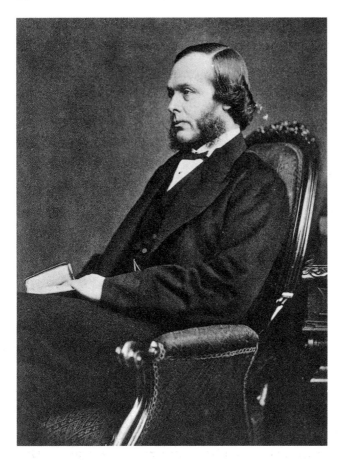

Fig. 4.2.
Lister, aged 42,
at the time he
left Glasgow for
Edinburgh, in
1869. (Godlee,
Lord Lister)

considerable detail, and the two stout volumes of the *Collected Papers* are good evidence of this. In January 1867 he began work on his report on the ten patients, and it was published in four instalments of *The Lancet* on 16, 23 and 30 March, and 27 April 1867. In the fourth instalment Lister was able to include an eleventh patient who had been admitted under his care on 4 April – a drunken man who had fallen from an open window and broken his right tibia and fibula. The unrestrained movements of his leg in the cab which brought him to the Infirmary resulted in drawing air into the tissues, which showed the crepitus of emphysema, and there was considerable loss of blood. Lister's house-surgeon, Dr Hector Cameron, having washed his hands and the leg in 1-in-20 carbolic lotion, squeezed blood and air from the leg, thoroughly swabbed out the wound with pure carbolic acid and splinted the whole limb. Recovery was enlivened by an attack of delirium tremens (treated with castor oil and morphine). However, by the time Lister corrected the proof of the last instalment in *The Lancet* on 27 April he was able to report that the patient was making good progress.

In July 1867 he published a fifth and final instalment, in which he described his method of providing safe drainage for cold (tuberculous) abscesses. These formed in patients with tuberculous disease of bones and joints – especially affecting the spine. If these were incised without antiseptic precautions they often acquired a secondary acute infection, with serious consequences. Lister found that if such an abscess was opened with sterile instruments, and dressed antiseptically, secondary infection was prevented, and the patient improved steadily, with healing of the wound.[14]

Lister had given careful thought to the title of this first report, which read: 'On a new method of treating compound fracture, abscess etc, with observations on the conditions of suppuration' (fig. 4.3). This, though strictly accurate, concentrated attention on compound fractures, which are not particularly common, and on carbolic acid as a dressing. Professor Syme recognised this difficulty and urged Lister to speak on the wider implications of antisepsis in an address to the British Medical Association Annual Meeting in Dublin in the following month. Here Lister spoke much more explicitly – 'On the Antiseptic Principle in the Practice of Surgery.'[15] He began by summarising the management of compound fractures:

the first principle must be the destruction of any septic germs which may have been introduced into the wound, either at the moment of the accident or during the time which has since elapsed. This is done by introducing the acid at full strength into all accessible recesses of the wound – then the mixture of clotted blood and acid, also any portions of tissue killed, are disposed of by absorption and organisation, *provided* they are always kept from decomposing.

In this way limbs which otherwise would be considered beyond salvage 'may be retained with confidence of the best results'.[16]

ON A

NEW METHOD OF TREATING COMPOUND FRACTURE, ABSCESS, ETC.

WITH OBSERVATIONS ON THE CONDITIONS OF SUPPURATION.

By JOSEPH LISTER, Esq., F.R.S.,

PROFESSOR OF SURGERY IN THE UNIVERSITY OF GLASGOW.

PART I.

ON COMPOUND FRACTURE.

THE frequency of disastrous consequences in compound fracture, contrasted with the complete immunity from danger to life or limb in simple fracture, is one of the most striking as well as melancholy facts in surgical practice.

If we inquire how it is that an external wound communicating with the seat of fracture leads to such grave results, we cannot but conclude that it is by inducing, through access of the atmosphere, decomposition of the blood which is effused in greater or less amount around the fragments and among the interstices of the tissues, and, losing by putrefaction its natural bland character, and assuming the properties of an acrid irritant, occasions both local and general disturbance.

We know that blood kept exposed to the air at the temperature of the body, in a vessel of glass or other material chemically inert, soon decomposes; and there is no reason to suppose that the living tissues surrounding a mass of extravasated blood could preserve it from being affected in a similar manner by the atmosphere. On the contrary, it may be ascertained as a matter of observation that, in a compound fracture, twenty-four hours after the accident the coloured serum which oozes from the wound is already distinctly tainted with the odour of decomposition, and during the next two or three days, before suppuration has set in, the smell of the effused fluids becomes more and more offensive.

This state of things is enough to account for all the bad consequences of the injury.

The pernicious influence of decomposing animal matter upon the tissues has probably been underrated, in consequence of the healthy state in which granulating sores remain in spite of a very offensive condition of their discharges. To argue from this, however, that fetid material would be innocuous in a recent wound would be to make a great mistake. The granulations being composed of an imperfect form of tissue, insen-

Fig. 4.3. The title page of Lister's first report on his first 11 patients, treated according to antiseptic principles. This report extended over five issues of *The Lancet* in 1867.

Lister then stated his belief that this encouraging success should be regarded as an illustration of a principle which could be widely applied: 'if severe forms of contused and lacerated wounds heal thus kindly under antiseptic treatment ... then its application to simple incised wounds – that is, deliberate operative wounds – must be a logical development.' Lister knew that his results had confirmed Pasteur's work, which had shown that air and surfaces of all kinds carried dust, which contained pathogenic micro-organisms. Therefore, if the surgeon's hands, instruments and drapes were soaked in 'a solution of carbolic acid in 20 parts of water – a mild and cleanly application – then it may be relied on for destroying any septic germs that may fall upon the wound during the performance of an operation.'[17]

This was a revolutionary concept at a time when, because of the threat of sepsis, a planned operation was only undertaken when the complaints of the patient compelled the surgeon to operate. In fact, Lister had felt justified in proceeding to practice elective surgery as early as 1866, when only four or five of the compound fracture patients had been treated. Eleven years later he described in a letter how he performed an osteotomy during the winter of 1865–66.[18] Hector Cameron also recalls two patients from this period with malunited fractures – one a severe ankle fracture, the other a fracture of the neck of the femur – that had united in so deformed a position that walking was not possible.[19] Lister removed his coat, rolled up his sleeves, and then 'the whole region of the operation, the hands of the operator and his assistants, and all the instruments, were thoroughly cleansed and immersed in a watery solution of carbolic acid'. Lister cut down on the region, refractured the bone with chisel and bone forceps, manipulated the limb to correct the deformity, closed the wound, and splinted the limb. 'All healed typically as antiseptic cases', and after some months the patients were 'able to walk firmly and well.'[20]

Then, in the summer of 1867, just after the publication of the first paper on compound fractures, Lister was presented with a real challenge to his belief in the role of antisepsis in surgery, when his sister, Isabella, consulted him. She had noticed a lump in her breast, and had already consulted James Paget in London, and Professor Syme, who both considered the lump to be cancerous, and too advanced to be operable. Lister, however, considered that an operation offered hope of relief, if not of cure. He proceeded to the dissecting room of the Anatomy Department in the University, to work out on the cadaver an approach which would include removal of the tumour and a full dissection of the lymph glands in the armpit – to which the cancer might already have spread. Thus prepared, Lister went over to Edinburgh to discuss the case with his father-in-law. Writing to his own father, Lister reported that Syme agreed that operation 'offered a chance, [with] the carbolic acid treatment depriving the operation of danger ... I felt his true kindness and manifest, though little expressed, sympathy very much, and left Edinburgh much relieved.'[21]

A room was cleared and prepared in Lister's own house, and there on 17 June 1867 the operation went ahead, with the assistance of Hector Cameron and two others. Later, Cameron recalled that 'those of us who assisted him saw how much it cost him to undertake so bold a procedure', and stated that he believed this to be the first time that this extended form of mastectomy had been successfully performed.[22] Isabella progressed well and there was no sign of infection in spite of the wide area exposed during the operation. She survived for three years, with no sign of local recurrence, but then succumbed to distant spread of the tumour.

This operation was the forerunner of the development, over the years, of 'kitchen table surgery', based on simple cleanliness and the immersion of scrubbed hands, instruments and drapes in dishes filled with 1-in-20 carbolic acid lotion. This basic routine, faithfully followed, was to be repeated over the next fifty to sixty years in palaces, houses, cottages, jungle hospitals and ships at sea all over the world. It was a safe and simple technique which could be followed anywhere, and it was pioneered by Lister's students and colleagues who had seen him at work in Glasgow and Edinburgh.

Over the next forty years Lister engaged in a steady flow of investigation, testing every aspect of the Antiseptic Principle. One of the best statements of this principle was made when, in 1875, he explored a knee joint in front of members of the British Medical Association at their annual meeting in Edinburgh. Operating and speaking in the surgical auditorium of the Surgical Hospital, Lister advised his audience that if digital exploration of the joint is required, it is necessary to

> take special care that it is an aseptic finger, cleansing it with antiseptic and making sure that it passes well into the skin around the nail. The chief essential for success is a thorough conviction of the presence of septic matter on all objects around us – you must be able to see with your mental eye the septic ferments as distinctly as we see flies with our corporeal eye ... if not you will be constantly liable to relax your precautions.[23]

It was unfortunate that Lister had taken some time before making it clear that the essential aim of antisepsis was to achieve the state of asepsis. Soon after 1875 surgeons began to boil their instruments, and referred to this as the 'aseptic' technique: this overlooked the fact that an aseptic operating technique had been achieved, using carbolic acid rather than heat, from the time eight or nine years previously when Lister first operated on malunited fractures, and on his sister Isabella.

Once he had made such striking deductions from his eleven patients, and devised a practical aseptic operating technique through the use of 1-in-20 carbolic acid lotion, Lister tackled the problem of stopping bleeding from divided blood vessels – which arises to some degree in all surgical operations. Thus far in the development of surgery, this problem had been approached by picking up a bleeding vessel with a forceps and throwing around it a ligature of silk or linen thread, which either lay in the theatre, or was kept threaded through the button hole of the operator's coat. This was then tied around the vessel and, the threads being left long, they were brought out through the end of the incision when it was closed. These ligatures were no more than outwardly clean so that in the interstices of the woven thread pathogenic germs lay, ready to develop in the wound and cause sepsis. To some extent the pus generated could escape alongside the threads, but sepsis around the ligature was proceeding, and the long ligature could only be withdrawn after 7–10 days, when suppuration had sufficiently weakened the vessel. If a firm clot had formed within the vessel, then withdrawal was uneventful, but often withdrawal disturbed a softened clot and then brisk 'secondary' haemorrhage ensued.

Experience with the antiseptic system led Lister to believe that 'if a silk or linen thread were steeped in a liquid calculated to destroy the germs in its interstices' and it was then tied around a vessel, and the ends of the ligature cut short near the knot, 'then it could be left with confidence that its presence would not ... occasion any disorder in the surrounding parts'.[24]

Lister's work on this subject began in December 1867, and introduces an important individual in Lister's life. This is Hector Cameron, already encountered as Lister's house surgeon earlier in that year. He had become a medical student in Glasgow in 1861, at the same time as Lister was taking up his position as Surgeon to the Royal Infirmary. At first Cameron would have been absorbed in pre-clinical studies at the University. However, it is likely that he would have heard stories about Lister, and would have walked up to the Infirmary building, stolen up the stairs of the Surgical Hospital, and entered the operating amphitheatre. There he would have watched Lister operate and been impressed by the personality of this thoughtful, modest, enthusiastic young man (Lister then being 34 years old). Cameron became a regular attender on Lister's ward rounds, and from 1865 he would have had the unique experience of watching Lister successively treat the patients involved in the trial of antisepsis in the management of compound fractures. Cameron graduated MB in 1866 and early in 1867 was delighted to become Lister's house surgeon (fig. 4.4). In this post he gained a wide experience, and later Lister was able to report that '15 cases of compound fracture were treated by my last house surgeon, Mr Hector Cameron, and every one of these men and women are living with their limbs on'.[25]

Lister recalled another occasion when in October 1867 a youth of 18 was admitted. In a fight, a knife with a 9-inch blade was thrust through his left rib cage below the armpit. Blood gushed forth and when the patient reached the Infirmary he was pale and shocked, and coughing up blood. The wound was still bleeding freely, and had a 5-inch length of omentum (the fatty apron in the abdomen) hanging from it, showing that the knife

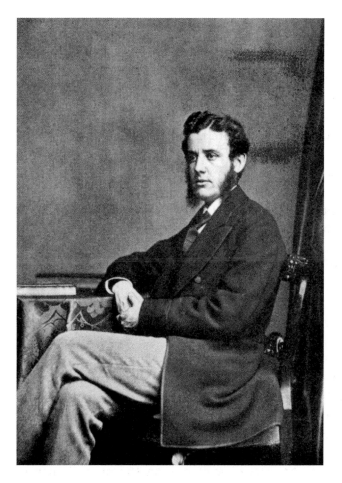

Fig. 4.4.
Hector Cameron,
aged 26, taken
towards the end
of his time as
Lister's assistant,
1867–69.
(Wellcome
Institute Library,
London)

had penetrated the diaphragm and entered the abdomen. At the time of admission, Cameron cut off the omentum and plugged the wound with lengths of lint soaked in carbolic acid in linseed oil, passing them in as far as possible. Bleeding gradually settled, and the patient improved until, after ten days, 'he was sitting up, singing songs, and conducting himself otherwise in an imprudent manner'. He had signs of fluid in the chest and several days of coughing up clots of blood, but after seven weeks he had healed and went home. Six weeks later, Dr Cameron saw him and another butcher in the street, 'driving an unruly herd of cattle, when our former patient, though pale, proved the more vigorous of the two, while his lusty exclamations, though not couched in the most decorous language, gave satisfactory evidence of the soundness of his lungs'.[26]

It is clear that a genuine friendship soon grew up between Lister and Cameron. Throughout his life Lister was reserved and found it difficult to make close friendships. Cameron was a warm, outgoing, supportive character, with wholehearted enthusiasm for Lister's pioneering work, and Lister came to appreciate and indeed to depend upon these qualities. At the end of Cameron's internship in late 1867 Lister invited him to become his assistant. Years later, Cameron's son, Charles, observed that 'my father was, I think, from the first aware that his unspoken belief in the marvel that was being wrought was in some way necessary and grateful to the man whom he venerated and obeyed'.[27] They formed a real partnership, working together until Lister left Glasgow two years later, and entered on a close friendship which endured for the rest of Lister's life.

One of their first collaborations was to investigate a safe method for the ligation of blood vessels, and in December of 1867 they went to the Veterinary College to operate on an old horse. Lister wished to test his belief that a ligature soaked in carbolic acid could be used to tie off an artery; then their threads could be cut off close to the knot and the wound closed. Operating with antiseptic precautions, and under general anaesthesia, they opened the left side of the neck, isolated the carotid artery, and tied it off with a length of purse silk which had been soaked in a strong watery solution of carbolic acid. The ends were cut short and the wound closed and dressed antiseptically: it healed cleanly. Six weeks later the horse died peacefully while sleeping in its stall. Lister was in bed at home with a severe cold, and Cameron was despatched by cab, with a supply of old towels, with instructions to cut out the block of tissue containing the operation area, and return with it, duly wrapped up, to Woodside Place. By the time that Cameron returned it was about 11 p.m. Lister rose from his bed and 'I could not dissuade him from proceeding to dissection', in the laboratory annex, which lasted until 2 a.m. The whole specimen was clean and the wound healed with 'the ligature still there, surrounded by healthy firm tissue'.[28]

Then in January 1868 Lister was asked to see a lady of 51 years with an aneurysm of the femoral artery 'as big as a large orange', situated just below the groin: it was very painful and prevented her from sleeping.[29] On 20 January, after steeping a silk thread in pure carbolic acid for two hours, Lister exposed the external iliac artery above the groin, tied it off and cut the threads short, near the reef knot. The wound healed cleanly, and six weeks later the patient was out walking, with the aneurysm both smaller and painless. Ten months later the patient died suddenly from rupture of an aneurysm of the aorta in the chest, and Lister was able to conduct an autopsy. He found the remnant of his ligature lying around the obliterated shrunken artery, above the aneurysm which had shrunk to the size of a cherry. Around the ligature was a cavity containing some opaque fluid: although there was no sepsis, this suggested to Lister that the threads of the ligature were causing some irritation, and this set him thinking of a suture material which, over some weeks, would be absorbed by the tissues. This led him to consider catgut, a possible candidate which, coming from animal tissue, is more likely to be absorbed by natural processes.

Commercially, catgut is made from the small intestines of sheep which are opened, cleansed, cut into ribbons, and stripped of some layers, leaving only the inner longitudinal muscle coat. These ribbons are then twisted to make threads of varying thickness. At Christmas 1868 Joseph and Agnes visited his parents at the family home in Upton, and there Lister made his first experiment with catgut. He converted his father's museum into an operating theatre, and there anaesthetised a young calf. The carotid artery was exposed in the neck and tied with 'minikin' fine catgut which had been soaked for four hours in carbolic acid lotion. Lister was assisted by his nephew, Rickman Godlee, then a student, who later, in his biography of Lister, recalled:

> I have a vivid recollection of the operation – the shaving and purification of the neck, the meticulous attention to every antiseptic detail, the dressing with a towel soaked in carbolized oil: and my grandfather's alabaster Buddha on the mantelpiece, contemplating with inscrutable gaze the services of beasts to men.[30]

A month later the calf was killed and Lister's father reported that the block of tissue had been removed and sent up to Lister in Glasgow, while 'the meat of the calf was divided up among the four men responsible, much I believe to their satisfaction'.[31] Lister was pleased to find that the catgut ligature – although looking unchanged – had in fact been invaded and replaced by living fibrous tissue. He made a detailed examination of this specimen and felt able to report that 'by applying a ligature of animal tissue antiseptically upon an artery, we virtually surround it with a ring of living tissue, and strengthen the vessel where we obstruct it'. This was a great advance on the use of a long unsterile ligature. Lister concluded: 'I would now without hesitation undertake ligature of the innominate (artery), believing that it would prove a very safe procedure.'[32]

In less than two months this statement received striking confirmation in a report from Mr Bickersteth, Surgeon to the Liverpool Royal Infirmary. He had operated on two patients, with enlarging aneurisms of the carotid and of the external iliac arteries, just three days after the publication of Lister's paper. Using catgut 'prepared according to the directions of Mr Lister', he had placed the ligatures to interrupt the arterial inflow into the two aneurisms, cut the ligatures short, near to the knot, and conducted the whole proceedings and aftercare under a 'strict antiseptic regime'. Both cases had healed cleanly, with excellent shrinkage of the aneurism. Bickersteth had been able to show both patients to James Paget, of St Bartholomew's, who was visiting, and who described them as 'brilliant results'.[33]

Lister's work on catgut was to continue throughout the rest of his life, with the last paper on this subject being written when he was 80.[34] As his knowledge grew he became aware of the variable behaviour of catgut, and a number of papers describe his experiments in the course of producing a truly reliable catgut suture and ligature. It remains his distinctive contribution that, in establishing the antiseptic principle, and the introduction of a safe absorbable ligature which could be cut short, he opened the way to modern surgical practice.

Although most surgeons continued, for some time, to regard Lister's results with scepticism, a few quickly recognised them as extraordinarily promising. In August 1868, just a year after his first papers, a report appeared in *The Lancet* from a surgeon quite unknown to Lister. Dr P. R. Cresswell, Chief Surgeon of the Dowlais Iron Works, Merthyr Tydfil, told how, over the past twelve months, the antiseptic system had 'created quite a revolution in his practice', which cared for over 8,500 workers.[35] He had treated wounds of every kind, and compound fractures, including a compound fracture of the neck and trochanter of the femur. Treated under antiseptic principles, this serious injury had healed soundly.

Visitors from Europe, who made rounds with Lister in Glasgow, also recognised the value of his work. Professor Saxtorph, from the old Frederick's Hospital in Copenhagen, was one of the first to spend time with him. Later he reported to Lister that, in contrast to previous experience, 'not a single case of pyaemia has occurred since I came home last year, certainly owing to the introduction of your antiseptic treatment. But it must be made clear to every surgeon that, unless you take the greatest precautions in *every* dressing till the wound is healed, you will never see the excellent results ... It takes longer and demands greater precautions, but the reward is certain.'[36]

Another early visitor, who became a lifelong friend, was Dr Just Lucas-Championnière from Paris, and it was he who, in 1876, published *Chirurgie Antiseptique*, the first book to provide a full account of the antiseptic system.[37] In the Introduction Lucas-Championnière recalled his visit to Glasgow in 1868 when 'I had the good fortune to appreciate antiseptic surgery almost from the very start ... I was so struck with what I saw that I made up my mind to do my best to make it known.' Later, in 1880, he wrote that 'we are in a position to do the most formidable operations, and that with the same security as if we were in the country, where the air is purest'.[38]

In spite of his growing reputation, especially in Europe, Lister remained modest, and in company a little unsure of himself, throughout his life. Cameron's son, Charles, remembered that at the age of 8 he was introduced to Lister, who was on a visit to his father. He was standing with his back to the fire, a cup of tea in his hand. Though by then a famous man, Lister had 'an indescribable air of gentleness and even shyness, but never awkward or ill at ease, and he moved with grace'.[39] Charles remembered country walks with his father and Lister, who still wore his tail coat and bow tie, and proved to be an authority on birdsong: Charles could not make the same claim for his father, who was however usually able to supply a good quotation from the poets.

Modesty and diffidence were shed when it came to work. Lister admitted that the prospect of a major operation always made him feel sick with anxiety, but once he had begun to operate nothing interfered with his concentration. He was certainly capable of decisive action in an emergency. Cameron tells of a morning when he was walking with Lister outside the Fever Hospital when they heard loud screams from a window on the second floor. Looking up they saw that a pane of glass had been broken, and a man was hanging out. He was suspended by one arm which was being held by a brave nurse. Lister dashed inside and up the stairs, two at a time. To gain access he grasped a poker and knocked out more of the glass. Then, taking another hold on the arm, he helped the nurse to hold on until porters arrived to rescue the patient.[40]

While development of the antiseptic system was absorbing much of Lister's time, and while he continued his heavy teaching programme and obligations to the University, there were major events arising in the family. In February 1869 Agnes's mother died, and then in April her father, Professor Syme, suffered a stroke. Agnes joined her sister Lucy in nursing her father, and Joseph often visited. Syme made a fairly complete recovery, but he recognised that at the age of nearly 70 it was time to retire from the Chair of Clinical Surgery.[41] Lister was already feeling uncertain of his future in Glasgow because in those days the rules of the Infirmary required the surgeons to retire after ten years' service: they then had to wait for a year before they could reapply for their position. The Edinburgh Chair, which his father-in-law had occupied for 37 years, was an attractive position, with security of tenure, and a less demanding teaching requirement. Lister submitted testimonials from James Paget and William Sharpey in London, E. R. Bickersteth in Liverpool, and Edward Lund – another disciple – in Manchester. Lister also received a letter signed by 127 Edinburgh medical students, who begged 'most respectfully to invite you to become a candidate for the Chair of Clinical Surgery, now rendered vacant by the resignation of our venerated teacher, Professor Syme. Your method of *Antiseptic Treatment* constitutes a well marked epoch in the history of British Surgery, and will result in unspeakable benefit to mankind.'[42]

Mindful of past misfortunes, Lister also re-applied for charge of his beds in Glasgow, which was not certain to go his way. However, this became unnecessary when, on 18 August 1869, he learned of his election to the Edinburgh Chair. This gave great pleasure to Lister's father, and to his father-in-law. His father, nearly 84 years old, was declining fast and Lister had to hurry down to Upton to be present when he died. From the time that he left home in his teens, Lister had written to his father most weeks and often at length, concerning every aspect of his life, and received equally regular and full replies. His father's own scientific outlook, as well as his solid paternal affection and support, albeit offered with Quakerly restraint, had been a constant support.

As he reflected on these events during his morning walks in Kelvingrove Park, during his last weeks in Glasgow, Lister must have welcomed the excavations and building going on just beyond the Park, on Gilmorehill (fig. 4.5). This was the site to which the University was preparing to move, from its centuries-old campus on the High Street. There its surroundings were 'dilapidated and overcrowded, including notorious slums. The College had been forced to abandon its evening law classes because each evening the air was thick with the human screams and policemen's rattles, while it was felt improper that students should have to walk to the College past a parade of prostitutes.'[43] In 1858, only two years before Lister began his lectures there, Commissioners to the University reported that 'the classrooms are small and low and their ventilation is bad. The College is surrounded with an atmosphere impregnated with the effluvia arising from the filth occasioned by such a population, in a town in which the sewerage is far from satisfactory, and with the fumes of chemical and other manufactories ... it is hardly possible to conceive of circumstances less favourable to the well-being of the youth attending a University.'[44]

Not only was the University moving to an open, hilltop site,

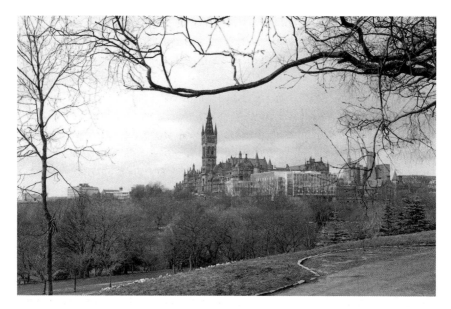

Fig. 4.5. The University of Glasgow buildings at Gilmorehill. Building work started in 1866 and was completed in 1887. (P.F.J.)

but the finance obtained from the sale of the old University site to the City of Glasgow Railway Company was sufficient to allow the building of a new teaching hospital, the Western Infirmary, beside the new campus. With the rapid growth of the population of the city there was an urgent need for such a facility, and the situation of the new Infirmary meant that the medical students would not have to make the long journey to the Royal Infirmary for their clinical work.[45] Lister, who had tolerated these conditions, must have been very appreciative of the advantages these moves would bring.

As his time in Glasgow was drawing to an end, Lister felt that he should draw attention to an unexpected but important effect which had followed the changes in treatment he had introduced over the previous four years. The paper was entitled 'The Effect of the Antiseptic System of Treatment upon the Salubrity of a Surgical Hospital'.[46] Lister had vivid memories of the state of the wards in the new Surgical Hospital which confronted him at the time of his appointment to Glasgow in 1861. 'This noble structure proved to be extremely unhealthy ... and my patients suffered from these evils in a way that was sickening and often heartrending, so as to make me sometimes feel it a questionable privilege to be connected with the institution.'[47]

Back in 1865, when Lister commenced his study of the antiseptic treatment of compound fractures, he was not thinking of its possible effect on ward hygiene. However, as confidence in the antiseptic regime grew, this encouraged him to test the underlying principle by introducing it into the conduct of elective operations, already described. By August 1867 he found that this gradual introduction of antisepsis into the routines of a whole surgical ward had such an effect that, over 'the last 9 months, not a single instance of pyaemia, hospital gangrene or erysipelas has occurred'.[48] This improvement continued over the following two years, 'although my wards have remained during 3 years without the annual cleaning thought to be essential'. When he asked the Superintendent the reason for this he was told that 'as those wards had continued healthy ... it had seemed unnecessary to disturb them'.[49] To this unexpected testimonial Lister could add his results in patients requiring an amputation: before antiseptic precautions there were 16 deaths among 35 patients (45%), but among 40 patients treated antiseptically there were 6 deaths (15%).'We have seen that a degree of salubrity equal to that of the best private houses has been obtained in particularly unhealthy wards of a very large hospital by simply enforcing strict attention to the antiseptic principle.' To avoid misunderstanding he went on to say: 'I mean not the mere use of an antiseptic, however potent, but such management of the case as shall effectually prevent the occurrence of putrefaction in the part concerned ... the same beneficent changes will take place when this principle is acted upon by the profession generally.'[50]

This approach revealed an aspect of Lister's character which did not help him to make his case. He knew that his careful work over the previous five years had given convincing proof of the truth of the antiseptic principle, and of its basis in the germ theory of putrefaction. His strong scientific background made it difficult for him to appreciate the slowness of most colleagues to adopt these principles. To bring his antiseptic practice to this point had required considerable courage, but this single-minded pursuit of the truth made him appear rigid and somewhat intolerant: he was always courteous, but perhaps gave the impression of self-righteousness. Here his shyness was a real handicap – a more relaxed and openly friendly man would have maintained warmer relations with colleagues, who would then have been the readier to consider the case he presented. It was right for Lister to report this unexpected and substantial improvement in the state of his wards, and for a meaningful report he had to compare it with the continued sepsis in other wards of the Infirmary. But it needed tactful handling.

Recently, some historians have suggested that these improvements in the state of Lister's wards, and those of his followers, were materially assisted by concomitant improvements in the social circumstances and nutrition of patients attending hospitals in Western Europe in the late nineteenth century. These must have been helpful, but they do not explain why adjacent wards within the Glasgow Infirmary should have been in so different a condition. Nor why Saxtorph and others who applied Lister's antiseptic principles should have seen so rapid a change in the incidence of sepsis in the wards of their hospitals.

Two weeks later *The Lancet* and the *Glasgow Daily Herald* carried a letter from the Secretary of the Infirmary which took strong exception to the contents of Lister's paper, and attempted to explain the 'satisfactory condition of the hospital' as being mainly due to 'the better ventilation, the improved dietary, and the excellent nursing to which the Directors have given so much attention'.[51] Lister replied courteously, but with a firm statement that changes in ventilation and diet could not explain the virtual disappearance of major sepsis from his wards. This was a sad ending to what had been a remarkable period in Lister's life, and he must have welcomed all the possibilities of his new post.

Many years later, in 1915, Cameron looked back to that time of controversy, and noted that 'it is a curious instance of "the whirligig of Time" that the present Managers consider the old connection with Lister the first feather in their cap, and proudly refer to it on all occasions.'[52]

CHAPTER FIVE

Development of the Antiseptic Principle, 1870–1880

Lister in Edinburgh

Joseph and Agnes Lister moved to Edinburgh in early October 1869. Travelling by train, they faced a 'perilous journey', with the famous four flasks of urine balanced on their knees, 'to the amusement of our fellow-travellers'.[1] They moved into the New Town, at first into temporary accommodation at 17 Abercrombie Place. It was only nine years since the Listers had left the city, and Lister was 42 years old as he took up his duties as Professor. Remembering his long wait to be appointed to the staff of the Infirmary in Glasgow, Lister had written in August to the managers of the Royal Infirmary of Edinburgh, saying that 'having been appointed Professor of Clinical Surgery in the University of Edinburgh, may I express the hope that you will provide me with the means of giving my lectures in connection with the Infirmary. Should you so honour me, the interests of the patients in my charge will be the primary object of my attention.'[2]

On 4 October the Managers gave their approval and allotted Lister the charge of fifty beds in the old Surgical Hospital – where he had previously worked as Syme's assistant. One of his colleagues there was Patrick Heron Watson who, back in 1854, had been one of the six dressers who had served Lister when he was Syme's house surgeon: Watson went on to be appointed Surgeon to the Royal Infirmary in 1860.

On 8 November Lister delivered his Inaugural Lecture as Clinical Professor, beginning with a tribute to his predecessor,

James Syme, who was present. 'Our old master is still among us, to aid us by his counsel, and his inexhaustible store of wisdom and experience.'[3] He went on to say:

> Clinical Surgery is surgery at the bedside, as opposed to surgery taught systematically in the classroom. The importance of bedside teaching cannot be overestimated, but is it possible to take a class the size of my present audience from bed to bed? Only a few can be thus taught. This difficulty was happily overcome by Mr Syme. It was easy in most cases to bring the patient before the class collected in the operating theatre, and hear not only the remarks of the teacher, but the patient's own account of the symptoms, and witness the treatment then and there put in practice. But you must not only see diseases but handle them and be personally concerned in their management, and these are supplied through the hospital offices of dresser, clerk and house surgeon.[4]

Several years later J. R. Leeson, who was a medical student at St Thomas' Hospital in London, was advised by one of the physicians – who had trained in Edinburgh – to pay a visit to Lister. Fifty years later he remembered his first impressions of the Surgical Hospital: 'A dark crowded stuffy building, smelling of distant carbolic, stale tobacco and ancient boiled beef'. The wards were crowded, often with 'shakedowns' on the floor between beds. However, there was 'sunshine within if little without' for he remembered 'the cheerful patients moving about, chatting to each other'.[5] As midday approached, there was a general bustle to tidy the wards and bring the carbolic sprays to readiness. Mrs Porter, one of the two senior nurses, would be to the fore, making sure all was right. She had worked with Syme for some twenty years, and was in charge of Lister's patients throughout the time that he was Professor. Some said he remained a little in awe of her. Leeson remembered the sound of Lister's landau, drawn by two bay horses, descending Infirmary Street, and rattling over the cobbles to the door of the Surgical Hospital. Lister would take the stairs two at a time, enter his small office at the turn of the staircase, and there meet his house surgeon and any visitors,

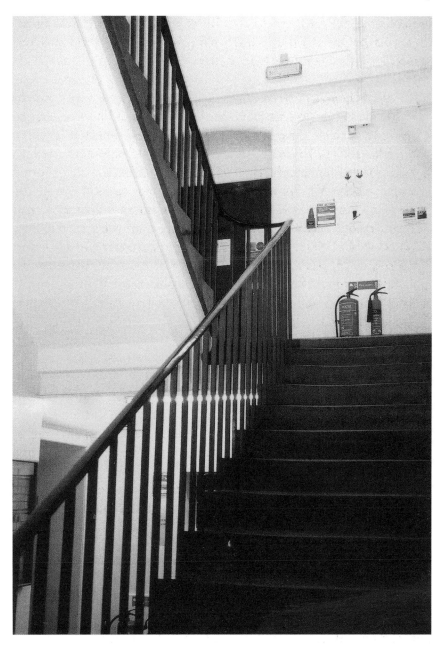

Fig. 5.1. The staircase in the entrance hall of the Surgical Hospital of 1832, in Edinburgh (see fig. 1.1). Lister used to run up the staircase, two steps at a time, to the room at the turn of the stair. Here Syme, and then Lister, met his house surgeon, any visitors from abroad, and interviewed new patients, such as Margaret Mathewson. (P.F.J.)

before starting the round of the wards[6] (fig. 5.1). All the post-operative patients had their wounds inspected, and those which showed no discharge on the bandage were left undisturbed. If there was any discharge, the dressing had to be changed. The spray was turned up, basins of 1-in-40 carbolic acid were brought – one for the instruments and one for washing the hands of the surgeon. Bandages were cut, the dressing carefully smelt, and the wound inspected. Drainage tubes might be shortened, then fresh dressings and bandages were applied. The pillows were adjusted and when Lister was satisfied that the patient was comfortable the bedclothes were replaced, putting them trim and square.[7] 'I had never seen such care bestowed on a patient, nor a surgeon working under such a sense of responsibility over a dressing.' Often Lister would say to his students: 'put yourself in the patient's place. What would you wish to be done were you in his case?'[8]

Leeson determined to become a dresser. There were twelve dressers on the firm, who fetched and carried and, from these, three students were chosen as clerks – they could take down selected dressings, and they kept detailed notes on each patient. Overall charge was in the hands of Lister's house surgeon, who was a graduate and held office for six months. Applicants for the position of dresser had to apply in person to Lister. Leeson remembered the visit to his house in Charlotte Square, when he was received with 'such a combination of refinement, ability, benevolence and sweetness of disposition'.[9] From that point he attended all Lister's rounds, and particularly recalled the Sunday afternoon visits. Lister would attend St John's Church in Princes Street in the morning, and then walk up to the Infirmary, where he made a ward round with his house surgeon, dressers and clerks.[10] In this relaxed atmosphere Lister became 'quite chatty'. He attracted the best students because he thought through every issue quite logically: knowledge was to be deduced from findings, not induced by rote. This led Lister on to explanations of the antiseptic system, and the reasons why he had to be so meticulous in all his work, because it was still on trial. This inspired a real sense of duty in everyone who worked with him, and this endured long afterwards in their own practice. One of Lister's strengths was his ability to make all his team – students and graduates alike – believe themselves to be his respected and appreciated colleagues.[11]

Lister welcomed the easier routine in Edinburgh, and was thankful that he did not have to lecture every morning at 08.30, but the days were just as full. 'In the mornings there were private patients to be seen, and operations to be performed. On the two lecture days in the week he liked to sit quietly thinking in his armchair, during which time he must not be disturbed. No other preparation was needed.'[12] The surgical amphitheatre had been built onto the back of the Surgical Hospital, and could seat 400 students, so it was large and lofty, with a big north window which illuminated the wide flat operating area. A semi-circle of old hair-stuffed chairs was provided for visitors. At 13.00 Lister entered and sat on an old chair, and then four dressers in blue check aprons brought in the patient, lying in a long wicker basket. The patient was greeted with a smile from Lister, and one of the clerks would present the case history. Lister would often question the patient to bring out salient points, and go on to demonstrate physical signs. The two or three patients shown would each illustrate some general principle, and sometimes the necessary operation would be performed there and then.[13]

In this event, three clerks were responsible, in rotation – one for the instruments, one to operate the spray, and one to administer the chloroform anaesthetic. The instrument clerk would already have the instruments ready on a tray, soaking in 1-in-40 carbolic lotion, and it had to be covered with a towel before being carried into the theatre. Lister required all his scalpels, once used, to be returned to the instrument-maker for resetting before they were used again, and his emotions if this were omitted were formidable.[14] He rightly believed that a truly sharp knife caused minimal damage to the tissues.

Chloroform was dripped onto a towel which was folded onto the face. Lister, an experienced anaesthetist, placed great emphasis on the importance of maintaining regular easy breathing: if it became difficult the towel was lifted and only air was breathed until regular breathing returned. This he considered to be much more important than observations of the pulse, because the respiratory centres were affected before cardiac functions.

The hands of the surgical team and the site of operation were thoroughly washed in 1-in-40 carbolic lotion, and then drapes soaked in the lotion were placed around the operation site and fixed with safety pins. By then the carbolic spray would be playing over the area and the operation could proceed. Bleeding points were picked up in forceps and tied off with catgut and the ligature cut short. Lister favoured leaving rubber tubes in the wound so that blood and serum did not accumulate and delay healing. Because anaesthesia allowed the surgeon to take time, Lister worked steadily rather that hastily, and by some was regarded as a slow operator. Forty years later, Godlee (his assistant for some years) commented: 'few if any of his students and assistants would have chosen any other surgeon to operate on themselves or their dearest friends. It was not only that sepsis would be avoided, but because they knew that the operation would be performed with a minimum of danger, and thoroughness impossible to excel.'[15]

There is no doubt that in operating before some 400 coughing, talking students, in a theatre which was rarely cleaned, Lister needed to exercise the full antiseptic ritual around the operating table. Soon after he moved to Edinburgh he introduced the idea of a spray which would diffuse a fine mist of carbolic acid over the table and the wound. Although he had obtained clean healing of his elective operation wounds in Glasgow by exercising great care over his antiseptic ritual, it is fair to say that he was haunted by the threat of sepsis. 'A floating germ might enter during the operation into some cellular interstice among the tissues and, becoming surrounded with a clot of blood, might escape the action of the antiseptic and, retaining its vitality, might subsequently propagate its kind, and spread putrefactive fermentation through the wound. But, by help of the spray, we operate in an antiseptic atmosphere and prevent organisms ever entering the wound alive.'[16] (It must be remembered that Lister had only a vague idea of the actual nature of germs at that time, and he can hardly be blamed for taking every precaution.) The spray gave Lister considerable peace of mind, for – 'the ideal is that carbolic acid should always be on outpost duty, and that the wound thus defended should be placed under conditions in which healing can proceed'[17] (fig 5.2).

From this time and for some fifteen years, at every operation and dressing of a wound, a spray would be operating. Many designs for spray-producing apparatus were evolved, some using steam generated in a water cylinder above a spirit lamp, while

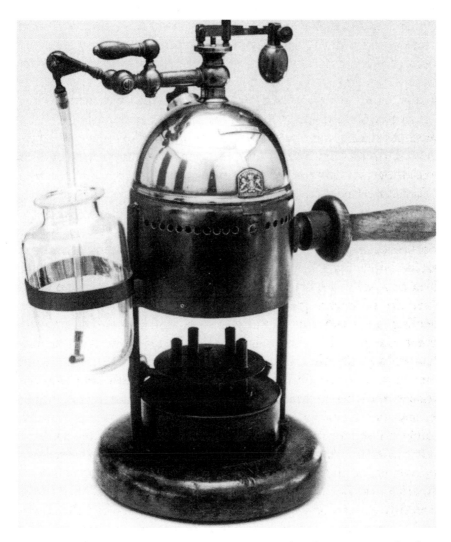

Fig. 5.2.   A Lister Steam Spray. Steam was generated in the main water chamber, which lies above the 5-wick spirit burner. The safety valve lies above the chamber. Steam passed along the horizontal pipe on the left. It absorbed 1-in-20 carbolic solution, siphoned from the glass jar beside the water chamber. (Pennington, T. H., *Scottish Medical Journal* 1988, 38: 218–19)

others used air compressed by a hand- or foot-operated pump. Steam or air under pressure was passed into a T-junction to which was attached a fine tube dipping into a flask containing 1-in-100 carbolic lotion. This fast-flowing stream of air or steam entrained a steady flow of the lotion, which emerged as a fine cloud of droplets. For some, who were sensitive to phenol, this could produce considerable discomfort, and everyone found the spray tiresome. However, great faith was placed in the 'unconscious caretaker'. Lister had secured excellent results in elective surgery before the spray was thought of, but in his anxiety he had considerably overestimated both the frequency with which air is contaminated by pathogenic germs, and the power of carbolic acid to annihilate them. By 1880 von Bruns in Tübingen suggested that the spray was not a useful element in the antiseptic system, and finally in 1887 Lister admitted that, 'I feel ashamed that I should ever have recommended it for the purpose of destroying the microbes of the air.'[18]

Shortly after its introduction the spray was brought into use for a distinguished patient. In 1870 Lister had been appointed Surgeon to the Queen in Scotland. All calls in this capacity remained strictly confidential, but some thirty years later Lister told this story to Hector Cameron's son Charles, who was a medical student in London.[19] In September 1871 Lister, who was on holiday with Agnes in Ambleside in the Lake District, received a telegram from Dr Marshall, who acted as Queen Victoria's physician when she stayed at Balmoral Castle. He sought Lister's help over the management of a painful abscess in the Queen's armpit. When Lister arrived on the following day, the Queen was clearly unwell, with a large acute abscess in the left armpit. Lister strongly advised drainage, and devised a spray by using a Richardson's atomiser, normally used for spraying local anaesthetic. Under a light chloroform anaesthetic (administered by the President of the Royal College of Physicians of Edinburgh), a deep axillary abscess was incised, with the carbolic spray providing cover, and a strip of lint was left in the wound as a drain. Next day the dressing was done satisfactorily, although at one stage the Queen learned of the disadvantages of the spray when Dr Marshall's grip on the apparatus slipped, and it was directed briefly into her face. Thirty-seven years later, in 1908 at the age of 80, Lister reported, quite anonymously, the progress of this operation.[20] 'Next day I found to my surprise on changing the dressing, that withdrawal of the lint was followed by the escape of thick pus. In that deep and narrow incision the lint acted like a plug.' After an anxious walk in the grounds, he decided to take a length of rubber tubing from the Richardson's spray. 'I cut holes in it, and attached knotted silk threads to the other end. This I put to steep overnight in a strong watery solution of carbolic acid [fig. 5.3]. Next morning I withdrew the lint dressing, when more pus drained, and introduced the rubber drain.' Following some further anxious perambulations, 'the next morning I was rejoiced to find nothing escaped except some drops of clear serum, and this rapidly diminished'.[21] The only indication in this paper of an unusual occasion was Lister's concluding remark that 'within a week of opening the abscess

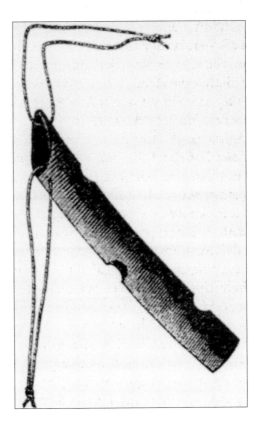

Fig. 5.3. Lister's drain. This is the pattern of rubber tube drain he devised for Queen Victoria at Balmoral. This design has been used by surgeons ever since. The thread is attached to a safety pin in the dressing. (Godlee, *Lord Lister*)

I was able to take leave of my patient'. There is an interesting footnote to this episode. As Lister was driven from Balmoral to Ballater station, he suddenly remembered that the tubing he had left in the wound was not secured by the safety pin which he always used. He had to admit his error, and bade the coachman drive back to the Castle. Here he offered his sincere apologies to the Queen, took down the dressing and inserted the vital safety pin. The Queen's comment on the whole affair was, 'a most disagreeable duty most pleasantly performed'.[22]

Another patient was Margaret Mathewson, aged 28, who in early 1877 came under Lister's care. She lived on Yell, one of the Shetland Islands, and had suffered from a painful left shoulder for a year. After a stay of eight months, she returned to Shetland, where she wrote of her experiences in a manuscript book entitled 'A Help to Memory'.[23]

During 1876 the arm had become progressively more painful and useless, and four months before admission an abscess at the swollen shoulder had been incised by the Parish Minister (there being no doctor on the island). This had left a discharging sinus, and it was decided that she should go to the Royal Infirmary in Edinburgh, with a letter of introduction from Rev James Barclay. When Margaret arrived at the gate and asked where she should go, the Gate Porter advised her to consult Professor Lister, in the Surgical Hospital. There she was met by Dr Watson Cheyne, Lister's house surgeon, who, by a happy chance, came from the neighbouring island of Fetlar, and knew Mr Barclay. He examined Margaret and advised her to wait, along with other patients, outside Lister's room. Lister asked her many questions about her shoulder, and about a cough which had troubled her for three years, and then examined her. Margaret remembered that 'Professor then sat down, folded his hands, and closed his eyes as if in silent prayer (which gave me more confidence in his skill). After a little he rose and came and felt it all over again', and explored the sinus with a silver probe.[24] He then turned to the students, commenting that the drainage of the abscess was good treatment, and said to Margaret: 'we will see what we can do for you'. Margaret was then escorted to the ward by Dr Cheyne, where she was glad to warm herself beside a large fire. 'There were 9 beds and all had nice white covers, clean pillow cases and sheets, and the room so tidy and neat.' She was welcomed by the staff nurse and encouraged to feel at home, 'for we are very homely and social here.'[25] (This orderly picture was unusual, and soon there were patients on beds made up on the floor.)

Patients were woken at 05.30 and helped in tidying the ward before breakfast was served – porridge and milk. Later gauze was torn into strips, and rolled to be used as bandages. Out-patients began to assemble from mid-morning, students arrived, and Professors Lister and Spence drove up at midday. Ward rounds commenced, and patients were chosen for teaching. Around one o'clock Lister went up to the theatre to operate, or to deliver one of his lectures, when patients would be examined and discussed. Patients who remained in the wards were served their dinner – soup followed by a dish of meat and potatoes. Margaret was sad to find that she missed her dinner when she was selected for teaching in the surgical amphitheatre. Here it seems to have been presumed that the technical language of the lecture would not be understood by the patient, but it was clear to Margaret that major surgery was being discussed and she became distressed. Lister saw this, patted her reassuringly on the arm, and turned her so that her back was to the audience. However, this gave her a view of the blackboard, on which was a chalk drawing of her shoulder, 'with special marks where it was to be operated on', and on seeing this 'I nearly fainted'. Dr Cheyne escorted Margaret back to the ward. Lister's words to the class probably covered the rationale of joint excision, and the great advantages it offered – if it proved successful – over amputation.

The pressure on theatre time was great, and in fact a fortnight went by, with a number of false starts, before she finally came to operation. At one o'clock Dr Cheyne came to escort Margaret up the crowded steps and into the theatre. There Lister bowed to her and smiled, and asked her to step on a chair and so onto the operating table. Chloroform was dropped onto a folded towel placed over her face and, 'I felt the professor's hand laid gently on my arm as if to let me know he was near me, and this did encourage me to hope for the best.'[26] Margaret then underwent an excision of the shoulder joint, which seems to have taken longer than usual, and she experienced quite severe post-operative vomiting. On the following day the dressing was changed by Lister, under the carbolic spray, with Margaret still troubled with sickness. Next day he came in to see her at 09.00, and 'seemed so glad, holding out his hand, saying "well, I am thankful to see you looking so well this morning. How are you?"' Margaret replied 'better but weak', and Lister said this was to be expected. 'He then folded his hands, closed his eyes in a short prayer, stood a few minutes thus bowed, and went out.'[27] A nine o'clock visit was unusual, and probably was a measure of Lister's very real anxieties over his patients, many of whom were receiving unorthodox treatment.

At first, passive movements of the shoulder were very painful, but Lister encouraged Margaret, and gradually she found she could move the arm. As her strength returned Margaret became well used to the routines of the ward. Patients woke early, had breakfast about 07.00, dinner around 13.00, tea with bread and butter about 16.30 and supper at 19.30, with milk and bread. Prayers were then said and the ward had settled down for the night by 20.30. Saturday evening was washing time, and on Tuesday and Friday the bed linen was changed, and the patients' personal clothes were washed.

Lister's last visit to Margaret was in September 1877, as he was leaving Edinburgh for London – this was some six months after the operation. He discussed her case with the students, and recalled that his first reaction to Margaret's condition was to advise amputation through the shoulder, 'but I thought again and again how I could save it, and at last concluded on excision of the shoulder as an experiment. Providentially, it has been a perfect success.' He asked Margaret to touch his hand, which lay on the bed, then to touch the pillow behind her head, and finally to touch her lips. 'This arm will be much more useful than one of wood or cork,' he said.[28] These patients, whose limbs had been preserved by joint excision, were a source of deep satisfaction to Lister. A month later, after several weeks at the Convalescent Hospital, Margaret returned home. In 1878, when Dr Cheyne came up to Fetlar on holiday, Margaret crossed over to see him, and reported that she could now do any sort of work around the house. Sadly, the tuberculous disease in her lungs again became active, and two years later she died from 'consumption of the lungs'.[29]

Margaret remained in hospital for eight months, and so long a stay was not unusual among Lister's patients with tuberculosis. The poet W. E. Henley came under his care in 1873, at the age of 24, when one leg had already been amputated below the knee. Finally, Lister had to amputate the other leg to control the disease, and Henley finally left hospital after a stay of 565 days. He survived until 1903, and recorded his memories of Lister in the *Cornhill Magazine* of May 1875:

> His brow spreads large and placid, and his eye
> Is deep and bright, with steady looks that still.
> Soft lines of tranquil thought his face fulfil –
> His face at once benign and proud and shy.
> If envy scout, if ignorance deny,
> His faultless patience, his unyielding will,
> Beautiful gentleness, and splendid skill,
> Innumerable gratitudes reply.
> His wise, rare smile is sweet with certainties,
> And seems in all his patients to compel
> Such love and faith as failure cannot quell.[30]

These very long admissions caused some problems for the managers, but Lister's explanations were accepted as reasonable. When he left Edinburgh, six long-term patients were accommodated for a time in private nursing homes, at Lister's expense.

Lister introduced several instruments which remain in active use. The humble sinus forceps, used in every hospital, looks exactly the same as its original, as do graduated steel urethral sounds. These are used for stretching up the long, narrowed male urethra which, in Lister's day and for long afterwards, often followed attacks of gonorrhoea. Inflammation would linger on, causing fibrosis with narrowing of the urethra until, in the 1940s, penicillin offered a rapid cure. These instruments still show the gentle curve in the shaft introduced by Syme, and the olive-shaped tip added by Lister. Until the mid-1950s every general hospital held a busy out-patient clinic for patients with chronic narrowing of the urethra who needed a regular dilatation. Lister, along with most surgeons, was well acquainted with the difficulties which could arise. He used his sounds with skill and gentleness – indeed, Leeson remembered Lister's unusual remark that 'no difficult stricture should ever be attempted unless the surgeon felt quite fit and, for example, had his bowels open that morning. Any little disharmony of his functions might detract from his delicacy of touch, and lead to failure.' He believed that, with few exceptions, 'if urine could get out instruments could get in'.[31] (Older surgeons still remember those days, and the apprehension with which the possessors of these difficult urinary channels would regard a new surgeon with his formidable instruments, who would be unfamiliar with their peculiarities. Although Lister's advice was not always followed to the letter, one rapidly learned that gentleness and great patience were essential elements in coping with the stricture clinic.)

In 1875 the Listers were probably enjoying the most satisfactory and fulfilling period of their life together. Agnes had the household well adjusted to the extreme variability of the time at which Joseph would return to see private patients, or take his meals. She was actively engaged in the much-needed social work of her church. In the evenings and well into the night Agnes would be willing scribe, technician and companion to Joseph in their laboratory. Here they had two main projects. Their notebooks are full of their trials to achieve a strong, supple catgut ligature; their work in bacteriology is best described in the next chapter. To offset these preoccupations, the Listers were good about organising interesting holidays together, in Britain, all parts of Europe and North America, when they became enthusiastic botanists.

Joseph found his wards constantly full, but with strict antiseptic precautions in theatre and at dressing-times, post-operative sepsis was well under control. At ward rounds visitors from home and abroad would often be present, and many became friends as well as converts.

When the British Medical Association visited Edinburgh for its annual meeting in 1875, Lister was able to report on a visit to Germany. Joseph and Agnes, with his brother Arthur and his family, first spent a month touring Italy, and then Joseph and Agnes went on for a month of visiting hospital centres in Germany.

In Munich Lister saw the great effect which the introduction of the antiseptic regime had produced – from a time when 80% of wounds became septic, 'they were doubtful whether they had one case of Pyaemia.'[32] They went on to Leipzig, Halle and Berlin, where they saw similar results, and Lister addressed the German Surgical Society. *The Lancet* commented: 'the progress of Professor Lister through the university towns of Germany has assumed the character of a triumphal march'.[33] In Munich 'Professor von Nussbaum was at the station on the morning of their arrival, in evening dress, with a large bouquet for Mrs Lister.' In Leipzig there was a 'Lister Banquet' attended by several hundred surgical staff and students. Professor Thiersch proposed Lister's health, saying: 'Lister's discovery, like other great discoveries, had to pass through the usual 3 stages – the first when the world smiles and says it is all nonsense: the second with a shrug and a look of contempt: and finally, "Oh that's an old story – we knew that long ago".' Lister replied in German, and then Professor Volkmann proposed the health of Mrs Lister. Songs in honour of Lister, set to student melodies, were sung by the whole company, and after many more toasts the proceedings ended after midnight.[34]

Their return to Edinburgh was most cordial. At his first student lecture there was a large attendance, and great cheering greeted Lister's entrance. The following year, in September 1876, Lister, Agnes and Arthur crossed the Atlantic in the *Scythia*, one of the last of the Cunarders to use both steam and sail, which allowed her to make 14–15 knots in a favourable wind. They landed in Quebec, visited Niagara and went on to Philadelphia, to an International Medical Congress attended by over 450 members. Lister was made President of the Surgical Section, and made a substantial address. This is said to have been received with close attention, with many questions, but generally his advocacy of the antiseptic system was received with considerable scepticism.

The party then took a round tour through the Rockies to San Francisco, and on the return journey they stopped in Chicago. Here they stayed with an old patient, from Lister's early days in Glasgow. A young millgirl sustained a severe injury to her hand while at work. This required a long period of treatment from Lister, but she was unable to return to fine manual work.

Lister persuaded her employer to give her a trial in the design department. This was so successful that eventually she was sent with samples of the firm's work to represent it at an international exhibition in Chicago. There she met a young American who was beginning in business; they married and became quite prosperous. When the patient learnt of the Listers' visit, she insisted that they should stay in her home.[35] The tour ended in Boston and New York, and the Listers were home by November. Work on the development of a sound catgut suture, and in bacteriology, was resumed, along with the full round of Lister's professional duties.

February 1877 saw an important change in Lister's affairs. On 10 February Sir William Fergusson died, and this initiated a train of events. He had been Professor of Clinical Surgery at King's College Hospital in London, but he had graduated and made his reputation in Edinburgh as a teacher of anatomy. In 1839 he joined the staff of the Edinburgh Royal Infirmary but only a year later was appointed to the chair at King's College in London. There he went on to establish a great reputation, and it was said that he had 'the eye of an eagle, the heart of a lion and the hand of a lady'.[36] He was not however an effective teacher, and the staff at King's had failed to attract students. Rather abruptly, only a week after his death, the *British Medical Journal* carried a news item to the effect that King's had to make some effort to compete with other teaching hospitals. (The physicians Richard Bright and Thomas Addison at Guy's, and surgeons like Liston at University College, James Paget at St Bartholomew's and Benjamin Brodie at St George's made a quintet whose reputation is still remembered.) The name of Lister was put forward as a candidate because 'Mr Lister's science and practice is now the most notable circumstance in British, or indeed European, surgery.'[37]

This news rapidly reached Edinburgh and at the end of his clinical lecture on 22 February Lister was presented with a vellum sheet signed by more that 700 students which began: 'We eagerly seize this occasion to acknowledge the deep debt of gratitude we owe for your clinical teaching ... many have gone forth, and many will still go forth, determined to carry your principles into practice ... we would yet earnestly hope that the day may never come when your name will cease to be associated with the Edinburgh Medical School.'[38] Lister replied in very warm terms and went on to say: 'there exists nothing in London which I consider good enough to call me away'. Continuing in this unfortunate strain, he compared the success of his lectures in Edinburgh with clinical teaching as he remembered it in London, which was conducted around the bed of the patient. This he suggested would be 'a mere sham'.[39] These remarks, so reminiscent of his condemnation of conditions in the Royal Infirmary in Glasgow were, not surprisingly, poorly received in London, and in March John Wood, already on the staff at King's, was appointed to the vacancy caused by Fergusson's death.

However, there were members of the staff at King's who felt that an opportunity had been missed; negotiations were reopened, and considerable efforts were made to meet Lister's requirements. In June 1877 he was appointed to a new Chair of Clinical Surgery.

Lister, mindful of his misjudgements, decided that it would be wise to take with him to London some assistants who knew his ways. First, he enrolled Dr Watson Cheyne, his house surgeon, who described how, one Sunday morning, he was asleep in his room when he was woken by Lister shaking him, to be invited to continue as his house surgeon in London.[40] Dr Cheyne needed no second invitation. He had come to Edinburgh from Shetland and one day, early in his student career, he was caught in the crowd sweeping into one of Lister's lectures. By the end of the lecture Cheyne was determined to become Lister's assistant. In the examination at the end of the course Cheyne was awarded Lister's prize, and he became a dresser. When he qualified Cheyne spent a year in the clinics of Vienna and Strasbourg. He was Lister's house surgeon in 1876, then his assistant, and eventually he himself became Surgeon to King's College Hospital. Dr John Stewart, a Canadian who was working with Lister, became the second member of the team.

William Dobie, a student, later described how in June 1877 he received a letter from Lister saying, 'I have no doubt by the end of the summer season you will be trustworthy in antiseptics. It would give me great pleasure to have you for one of my dressers.'[41] James Aitken, another student, made up the quartet bound for

King's: they were to be fully employed over the coming months, and were to share many difficult experiences.

Rickman Godlee, in his biography of his uncle, commented, 'Lister never forgot the debt which he owed to Edinburgh. No place in the British Isles could have provided him with such a class, or such good opportunities for pathological or clinical research, or for spreading his influence among foreigners.'[42] However, as Godlee continued, 'Lister was now a man with a mission. The antiseptic doctrine had been accepted in every part of the world that counted, except London, where alone it made little headway. The importance of converting the greatest centre of learning and education in England justified almost any sacrifice.' He must 'let them see how he actually carried out the treatment himself, and the results he was able to obtain'.[43]

Ogston in Aberdeen

One of the first visitors to Lister, following his return to Edinburgh from Glasgow in September 1869, was a young surgeon from Aberdeen, Alexander Ogston. Born in 1844, the son of the Professor of Materia Medica, he entered the University of Aberdeen, aged 15, at first joining the Arts Faculty and then going on to read medicine. At the age of 18 he was a student in the wards of the Aberdeen Royal Infirmary where conditions there and in the operating theatre must have been daunting and troubling.[44] Then in 1863–64 Ogston took a year out, to visit the main teaching centres in Central Europe. His memories of Prague were chiefly of the ferocity of the bedbugs; Vienna he remembered for its beauty, and atmosphere, and the many friends he made among the hospitable student community – with great benefit to his command of German. In Berlin the social scene was distinctly cooler, but Ogston found it a more interesting and lively medical centre. He was particularly inspired by two professors – Langenbeck and von Graefe. Langenbeck was the leading surgeon, and later in life Ogston placed him alongside Lister for his personal character, and devotion to the development of surgery. Langenbeck was the founder of the Congress of German Surgeons where, later, Ogston was to benefit greatly from its tradition of granting a fair hearing to new ideas. In the Ophthalmic Clinic von Graefe was outstanding for the kindness and courtesy he showed to everyone, and for the developments he was making in ophthalmology.[45]

Back in Aberdeen, Ogston graduated with honours in 1865, and spent some time in general practice. In 1866 he opened an eye dispensary in the city, in which he worked until 1868 – his time with von Graefe had proved fruitful. In September 1868 the ophthalmic surgeon to the Infirmary, J. R. Wolfe, left for Glasgow and Ogston, aged 24, was appointed to fill the vacancy. In the following year the register shows that 102 ophthalmic operations were performed, 16 for cataract.[46] In view of the conditions in the theatre, it seems likely that some of these procedures would have become septic. His long experience of the frequency of post-operative wound infection must have left him particularly ready to learn 'with incredulity, that Lister had discovered a means of avoiding suppuration'.[47]

Ogston 'resolved to go and see', and in October 1869 he went to Edinburgh. There, 'without any introduction, I called on Lister at his own house and was received, though unknown, with all the sweetness and courtesy which was a part of his nature … we had a long talk.'[48] Lister had just moved from Glasgow, to take up the Chair of Clinical Surgery, and had barely commenced his clinical duties: he advised Ogston to visit Hector Cameron who was continuing his work in Glasgow. Cameron was fortunate to have beds in the wards of Lister's successor, Professor George Macleod, who was himself a convert to antiseptic surgery. Cameron took Ogston to visit his patients: 'Five minutes later found me convinced – I was shown a knee joint which had been opened, and was allowed to handle it. There could be no room for doubt. Where was the inflammation? The limb was perfectly well, and I was shown other cases. I saw that a miraculous change had come over our science … and inclined to think out what the great revelation implied for the future.'[49]

Ogston returned to Aberdeen, and 'from that time I introduced the methods of Lister'. The managers complained of the cost of providing fresh dressings and lotions for each patient, and 'older members of staff were indifferent, if not actively hostile', but from then on Ogston always followed Listerian principles. In the following year, 1870, at the age of 26, he was appointed Junior Surgeon to the Royal Infirmary. The duties were light – only 74 general surgical operations were performed in the whole of that year – and he was able to fulfil the duties of Assistant Chloroformist, and Aural [Ear] Surgeon. Throughout the 1870s the number of operations performed annually did not exceed 150: so real had been the threat of post-operative wound infection that surgeons were accustomed to operating on a very limited range of conditions. Even though an effective antiseptic regime had become available, it was difficult to consider widening the field.

It was here that Ogston was one of the first to give a lead, following Lister's venture of the mid-1860s into the field of elective operations on bones. In 1874 Ogston became Full Surgeon and was free to make his own decisions on the patients under his care (fig. 5.4). He must have been familiar with the many children who hobbled about Aberdeen, handicapped by their knock-knees or bowed legs. These were due to rickets,* which impaired the ossification of developing bones: so, as weight on the legs increased these deformities could develop. The pioneer operation for knock-knee was performed by Thomas Annandale in Edinburgh in March 1875. Ogston felt that this caused too much damage to the articular surfaces of the knee, and he devised a more conservative operation.

His first patient, a lad of 18, had bilateral knock-knee (genu valgum) which had developed over ten years. 'When he walks he drags the posterior knee from behind its fellow, makes it circumnavigate the latter, and finally come in front of it, before the weight of the body is transferred from one limb to the other.' Figure 5.8 (p. 137) shows the deformity and the principle of

---

* Rickets is now known to be due to a deficiency of vitamin D, occurring in dairy products, and synthesised in the skin when regularly exposed to sunlight. These were largely denied to children receiving a poor diet, and rarely seeing the sun as they played down shadowy city wynds and closes. James Maxton, the future Labour MP, recalled that when he taught 'a class of 60 boys and girls of about 11 years old, 36 of the 60 could not bring both knees and heels together because of rickety malformations.'[50]

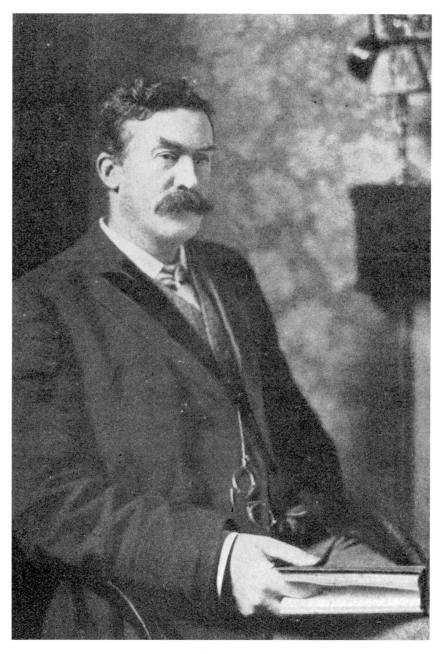

Fig. 5.4. Professor Alexander Ogston, aged 52, in 1896. (Ogston, W. H., ed., *Alexander Ogston*)

Ogston's operation, which allowed the detached elongated inner condyle of the femur to slide upwards into a normal position. On 17 May 1876, under chloroform anaesthesia, 'the whole operation was conducted under carbolic spray, with a minute observance of Lister's antiseptic precautions'.[51] Through an incision on the inner side of the left knee, a saw was inserted, the cut almost completely detaching the left condyle from the femur. The lower limb was then grasped and firmly brought inwards, at the level of the knee: the pressure upwards from the inner tibial condyle forced the detached condyle up into its proper position. The incision was closed and an antiseptic dressing applied. The straightened limb was kept splinted for some weeks and recovery was uneventful. On 6 June the right leg was similarly corrected. The patient was allowed to walk on 9 July, and he left hospital 'walking perfectly' on 21 July.[52]

Like Lister, Ogston was performing an unorthodox operation surrounded by critical observers. He had the added anxiety of having to work in a dusty ill-ventilated theatre, crowded with interested students, and used by other surgeons who did not observe antiseptic precautions. It is understandable that he should take such care over his antiseptic precautions. The first detailed account of this operation appeared in the *Edinburgh Medical Journal* of March 1877.[53] The following month Ogston attended the annual Congress of German Surgeons in Berlin, and described his operation, with subsequent publication in the *German Archives of Clinical Surgery*.[54] This led to his operation becoming widely known in Europe. It was certainly an advance on Allandale's procedure, and prepared the way for Macewen's. By 1878 antiseptic osteotomy was well established in Britain and in Europe as a safe operation with great long-term benefits for the patient.[55]

Lister's belief, based on the work of Pasteur, was that wound infection occurred when germs carried on dust alighted on an intentional or accidental wound in the skin. He did not, at this stage, have any objective evidence of the nature of these germs, but Ogston went a step further: 'often I meditated on this subject and became convinced that there was a single cause, and that the cause was some special germ'.[56] It may well be that his thoughts were further stimulated by a visit to the Congress of German Surgeons in April 1878. This was primarily to hear two papers on the results of the Ogston operation, but there was the additional attraction that Theodor Kocher, Professor of Surgery in Berne, was to speak on 'The Aetiology of Acute Infections': it seems more than likely that Ogston would have met Kocher to discuss this topic.

Stimulated by these contacts and by reading the 1877 paper of Robert Koch, the German pathologist, on the staining and microscopy of bacterial specimens,[57] Ogston embarked in the summer of 1878 on a long study. This was to establish him as a leading figure in the developing science of bacteriology. 'It started one day when I had to attend a young man suffering from an extensive abscess of the leg. Procuring a clean phial, I evacuated into it the matter through the unbroken skin, proceeded home with it and placed a little of the pus under an ordinary student's microscope. My delight may be conceived when there were revealed beautiful tangles, tufts and chains of round organisms in great numbers, which stood out clear and distinct among the pus cells, all stained with aniline violet solution.'[58] Ogston checked these findings by examining pus from every abscess opened by him and his colleagues. In 65 acute abscesses he found micrococci in abundance, some arranged in chains, and many in clusters, like grapes.

In September 1878 Koch published his book on *The Aetiology of Traumatic Infective Diseases*, which gave details of staining techniques, and stressed the importance of using a microscope with an Abbe condenser and a Zeiss oil immersion lens. These only became available in January 1879, and Ogston must have been one of the first to purchase this equipment, with a grant from the Scientific Grants Committee of the British Medical Association. Foreseeing the need for an extensive investigation, he built a hut in the garden of his house, 252 Union Street, Aberdeen, and installed his new apparatus there, with an incubator, and cages for small animals. He obtained a licence allowing experimentation on animals.[59]

'Using the methods of Koch, which I followed exactly',[60] Ogston found that when he injected a drop of pus from an acute abscess under the skin of a guinea pig or a mouse, it became ill, and micrococci appeared in the blood. Sometimes this went on to septicaemia and the animal died, in others the bacteraemia resolved and an acute abscess formed at the site of the injection. Pus from such an abscess, if injected into another animal, produced the same sequence of disease, but pus heated or treated with phenol had no effect: Ogston concluded that it must have been living organisms which had produced an abscess.[61] At this stage he extended the range of his investigations and found innumerable cocci arranged in chains in the vaginal discharges of patients with puerperal fever, and cocci arranged in bunches from patients with acute osteomyelitis (infection of long bones) (fig. 5.5).

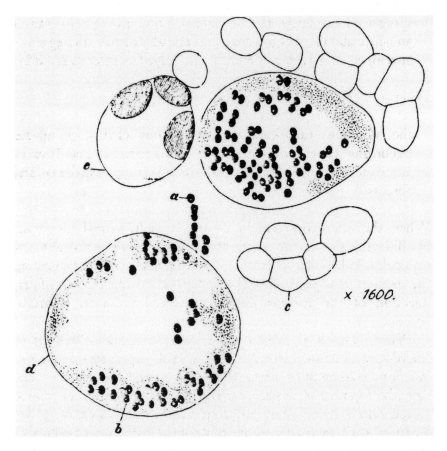

Fig. 5.5.   Photomicrograph of micrococci in extravasated blood, drawn in 1880 by Ogston to illustrate his article in the *Archiv für Klinische Chirurgie*.

However, after many observations on urine and blood specimens, taken from healthy people, Ogston stated the important negative finding that micrococci do not exist within the tissues of healthy people, although they abound on the surface of the skin.

Ogston then wished to grow micrococci in pure culture, to find out whether an injection of the germs alone would reproduce the same signs of disease. In 1879 there was no reliable way of growing micro-organisms in the laboratory, and Ogston made many inconclusive experiments using urine and other body fluids as a culture medium.

> Finally I hit on the idea of growing them in eggs. Newly laid eggs were washed in 5% carbolic water, and under the carbolic spray a minute aperture was pierced – one minim of pus from an acute abscess was injected into the albumen ... the egg was enveloped in a Lister's dressing and kept for 10 days at 98°F.

When the egg was opened,

> the albumen was filled with enormous chains or masses (according to the coccus used) of micrococci ... a drop of albumen injected into an animal's back now produced a typical abscess.[62]

When the micrococci lay in chains (already named *streptococci* by Billroth) the infection produced was severe, with signs of erysipelas. When the cocci grew in clumps like grapes (suggesting the name of *staphylococcus* to the Professor of Greek in Aberdeen) injection of the culture usually produced an acute localised abscess.

When Ogston presented these results to his colleagues in Aberdeen he was surprised by their general scepticism – immersed in a large volume of evidence which had provided incontrovertible facts, he found this rigidity extraordinary. In London he visited Lister, now a firm friend, and found him much more receptive. Then in April 1880 Ogston again attended the annual meeting of the Congress of German Surgeons, and spoke of his researches in a paper entitled 'Ueber Abscesse'. It was received with acclamation and he was elected a Fellow of the Society.[63]

In 1881 Ogston reported to the Scientific Grants Committee of the British Medical Association which had helped him to set up his laboratory. Reading this report now, one is impressed by the sheer volume and detail of the observations which were made.[64] Ogston writes as an experienced pathologist, quite familiar with the practicalities of microscopy, staining techniques and the care of small animals. It is a remarkable document when it is remembered that it was produced in a garden shed, by a general surgeon, at a time when there was only a handful of workers interested in bacteriology. Now, Ogston is accepted as the discoverer of *Staphylococcus aureus*: he was 'the man who correctly interpreted the exact aetiology of acute suppurative processes in man'.[65]

In the following year, 1882, Ogston became the Regius Professor of Surgery in Aberdeen. With daily lectures and obligations in the university, and a widening range of surgery in the infirmary, he made no further observations in his laboratory. He was a tall, imposing figure who left a strong impression on his students as a good lecturer, and in the wards they remembered the courtesy and consideration with which he met each patient. Bedside teaching was still vital: accurate determination of physical signs was essential, especially before the arrival of X-rays. However, the students' memories of the crowded operating theatre at the top of the Simpson building seem rather clouded in the mists of the carbolic spray.

Very little is known of Ogston's two wives (the first died when young) but their large family write warmly in their memoir of their father.[66] Although a busy and rather remote figure, he emerged for birthdays and festivals, and they all had good summer holidays as they roamed and cycled from their holiday house in Upper Deeside. They speak – especially the girls – of the warmth of his understanding and support as they grew up. Alex Ogston had a long life and it proved to be full of interest.

In 1882, the year of his appointment as Professor, Ogston made his final report on his laboratory work. The sceptical editor of the *British Medical Journal*, on this occasion, declined to publish it. Mindful of the prevailing opinion, Ogston submitted his paper elsewhere, and concluded with these forceful words:

> The present is an epoch in which it seems somewhat unfashionable to be a thorough antiseptician in theory and in practice, when such words as bacteria and carbolic acid have become commonplace and vulgar. Human nature forgets unseen foes, but if every physician and surgeon were familiar with the microscopic study of microorganisms then, beholding both our faults and their punishment in the treatment of wounds and disease, it would be less easy for fashion to mislead, or prejudice to warp, our minds.[67]

Macewen in Glasgow

When in the autumn of 1869 Ogston travelled to Glasgow to meet Hector Cameron, and visited his patients in the Surgical Hospital of the Royal Infirmary, he may have met William Macewen. Cameron cared for his patients in the wards of Professor George Macleod, and William Macewen, who had just graduated, was Macleod's house-surgeon.

Born in 1848, on the island of Bute, the youngest of twelve children, Macewen as a youth was 'tall and full of vitality, intelligent but indifferent to books, more at home in the gymnasium than the classroom'.[68] As a child he had spent much time with the skilled workmen of a local boatbuilding yard, who taught him the right use of tools. In time, he decided to study medicine and entered the University of Glasgow in the autumn of 1865, at the age of 17. In 1867 he began to attend Lister's ward rounds, just as Lister was completing the series of patients with compound fractures, whose results provided the basis of the antiseptic system. Many years later, Macewen spoke of the privilege of being a student of Lister:

> to be allowed to watch the habit of mind, and see how the brain worked. He was a man in earnest and therefore he taught. He accumulated data by observation and experiment, from which careful deductions were drawn. He laid bare the difficulties

he encountered, and his modes of overcoming them, and so stimulated the thinking of the student – and paved the way for others to follow.[69]

This must have made a strong impression, for Macewen was not a man to be impressed by received opinion or by authority, however distinguished.

At the end of his life, when seriously ill, Macewen was visited by a close friend who tells how, quite suddenly and in a quiet voice, Macewen spoke of his early days as a student.[70] Once, when the sights, smells, sounds and suffering of the hospital proved unbearable, Macewen sought out a seat in the fresh air, 'to consider whether he could continue a study which could show only such results'. An elderly woman of the domestic staff was passing, as he sat in gloomy contemplation. She stopped and said 'What's makin' ye sae sad the day, laddie?' To which he answered with a wave of the hand to the hospital, 'Who could help being sad at these things?' The woman replied that 'it would be to more purpose to go back and try to mend them'. Macewen returned to the ward and was examining a recent amputation stump, with the long ligatures still hanging from the wound: 'they looked dirty'. He went to the empty operating theatre and looked at the unused ligatures, made of hemp and kept in a jar, and they did not seem clean. He then sought permission,

> to try if boiling would improve them, and from the ligatures he passed to the needles and on to the instruments, with increasingly appreciable results: but he could not secure the cleanness of the hands of the attendant who handled them all ... it was as if the speaker's mind travelled back down the long trail and saw, far down amid the darkness, ignorance and pestilence, the very spot and moment from which he had deliberately set forth on a determined road.[71]

As a young graduate Macewen had no savings, and in 1870 he worked for a year in the Glasgow City Fever Hospital. Built in 1865, with separate pavilions of wood built on brick foundations, it was the first municipal hospital in Scotland for fever patients. Here

Macewen saw the desperate state of some children with diphtheria – then a common infectious disease. The membrane which formed in the throat could spread down to the vocal cords, causing narrowing of the airway, and this could choke the patient. At that time (and for long afterwards) this was relieved by the operation of tracheostomy – an incision was made into the windpipe below the vocal cords through which a tube was passed, allowing free breathing. This remained until the membrane cleared away. (The writer remembers that in the 1930s the mother of a school friend was seriously ill with diphtheria. She had to have this operation performed in the middle of the night, in her bed, in her own home, by our general practitioner. To give her peace and rest, hay was laid down on the street outside to quieten the sounds of horses' hooves and the iron tyres of the carts they drew, until she recovered.) It occurred to Macewen that it might be possible to pass a tube through the mouth, between the thickened vocal cords, into the trachea, and so relieve the obstruction. This would avoid the real dangers of an open operation on the neck. He adapted rubber and gum-elastic catheters and, using himself and bodies in the mortuary as subjects, he found that a tube could be passed over the back of the tongue, using the left forefinger to depress the epiglottis, and to guide the tube between the cords. This was a considerable advance, and when Macewen reported his experience in the *Glasgow Medical Journal* it attracted much attention and the article was translated into French. He anticipated by many years the introduction of tracheal intubation in the practice of anaesthesia.[72]

In 1871, at the age of 23, Macewen was appointed medical officer to the Glasgow Poor Law hospital, known as the Town's Hospital. Here in fairly basic conditions he began operating on hernias in the groin (patients were kept in bed for 4–6 weeks!). Working with the Superintendent, Dr Robertson, Macewen also began his long study of the operative treatment of mastoid infection secondary to chronic middle ear disease.

In 1873 Elizabeth, aged 29, was admitted under Macewen's care complaining of abdominal swelling which had become increasingly painful. Her appetite was poor and she often vomited. Walking was difficult owing to the size of the swelling. Examination showed pallor and emaciation, with rapid uneasy breathing and signs typical of a large ovarian cyst. Although very much aware of the risks, Macewen felt that the cyst should be removed, and the patient 'eagerly begged' that this should be done.[73] Even so, in 1873 abdominal operations were rarely performed. Both Wells and Keith had reported in 1869 and 1870 on their results in ovarian cystectomy, but with their considerable experience they still had a mortality rate of around 20%. It was a major responsibility for a young man, only four years qualified and relatively inexperienced, to take on such a case, especially when he had decided to adopt an unorthodox technique. Surgeons had great reserves over leaving the ligated stalk of an ovarian cyst to shrink within the abdomen, where it could become a focus for infection, and Wells and Keith were still leaving the stalk long, held out in a clamp, on the abdominal wall. Macewen was certainly concerned about this, but he believed that if the stalk of the cyst was tied off with sterile catgut, which was absorbable, it could be cut short and safely left deep within the abdomen.

Lister was working on the preparation of catgut ligatures in 1868, while Macewen was still a student, and in his 1869 paper Lister gave details 'for surgeons who may wish to prepare it for themselves'.[74] By 1873 Macewen was also experimenting with catgut and he had probably prepared the catgut which he wished to use when he operated on Elizabeth. However, before proceeding, he felt that he needed another opinion, and decided to write to Lister in Edinburgh for his advice. Many years later, Macewen's son John revealed the story which his father had told him about this request.[75] Macewen waited in vain for a reply, and finally decided to trust his own judgement, and to proceed to operation on 30 September 1873.

A single well-lighted and ventilated room was obtained, and its temperature regulated at about 65°F. The patient was bathed and dressed in clean clothes whilst 'care was taken to have the person and clothing of the staff properly fresh and clean ... a carbolized atmosphere was provided by the carbolic spray, instruments, sponges and hands of the operator and assistants were bathed in heated carbolized solutions.'[76] Through a midline incision the cyst was exposed and evacuated, when hundreds of rounded pellets were discharged. Then the cyst was delivered and adhesions to the omentum divided ... 'The pedicle [stem of the cyst] was short, broad and highly vascular, and an encircling catgut ligature did not control the bleeding. The pedicle was therefore transfixed in 3 places and secured by 4 antiseptic catgut sutures.'[77] The abdomen was carefully sponged out, the short stalk of the cyst inspected and found to be dry, and so was dropped back into the abdomen. The incision was closed with deep catgut sutures embracing all layers of the abdominal wall.

John Macewen then resumed his account: 'On his return from the operation my father found Lister's answer awaiting him. Written from Lyme Regis where he was on holiday, Lister apologised for the delay in replying: 'I am not prepared to advise the use of catgut for the pedicle in ovariotomy', and went on to discuss alternative solutions.[78] 'My father had several days of misery in consequence until, the case going well, he realised the delay had been a blessing in disguise.'[79] His concerns were understandable because Elizabeth was a significant operative risk: with a large cyst she was likely to be under-nourished and anaemic. Maintaining fluid intake after operation was always a problem before the advent of intravenous fluids, but frequent sips of water, ice and beef tea were given. A rectal tube was used to relieve flatus, and also to administer beef tea and eggs! It was a week before the patient was passing wind spontaneously per rectum and taking some food. The wound healed well but 'she was kept in bed for 4 weeks, though latterly clamorous to get up. Now, 8 weeks after operation, quite able to walk freely, though still weak.'[80]

A week after the operation Macewen wrote to his brother-in-law, Dr James Allan, who had been his close friend through childhood and college days. He tells of his concerns during the operation and afterwards and concludes, 'I doubt she will die, but she won't if I can help it.' Then he adds, 'Mary Ann is an angel'[81] – a reference to Mary Ann Allan, his wife of a few months' duration. Subsequently all too little is heard of Mary Ann, who gave William and their six children tremendous support throughout their lives. Three sons qualified in medicine, and John followed his father as Surgeon to the Royal Infirmary of

Glasgow.

In 1871 Macewen was also appointed Casualty Surgeon to the Central Police Division of Glasgow, a position which provided a wealth of surgical experience, especially at the week-ends. Here he made useful observations on the behaviour of the pupil of the eye in alcoholic stupor, abdominal injuries and the right use of the stomach tube.

Macewen was elected to the staff of the Royal Infirmary in 1874, and 2 years later, at the age of 28, he became Full Surgeon, with charge of wards (fig. 5.6). These – wards 21, 22, and 29 – left a good deal to be desired, being situated in the old Fever Hospital. The operating theatre – described as 'wretched' – needed thorough cleaning and reorganisation, and was equipped with a

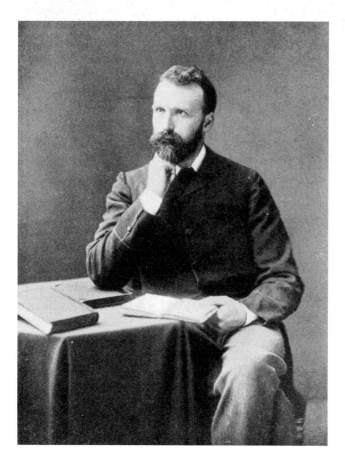

Fig. 5.6. William Macewen in 1876, aged 30. (Wellcome Institute Library, London)

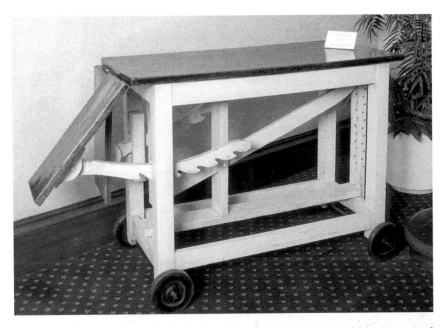

Fig. 5.7. Macewen's wooden operating table. (Royal College of Physicians and Surgeons, Glasgow)

solid wooden operating table made to Macewen's design (fig. 5.7). For the time being he adhered to strict antiseptic precautions, which enabled this theatre to be the site of some remarkable developments.

Charles Cameron remembered from his childhood how 'throughout the city the pinched faces and misshapen bodies of the poor were everywhere to be seen.'[82] Macewen was very much aware of the problem – 'Rickets is one of the most widespread diseases incidental to large manufacturing communities, such as London, Manchester, Glasgow and Lyons. Jenner describes it as very abundant among the London poor: Delore says that no sooner is a hospital ward opened in Lyons for the cases of rickets than it is filled to overflowing: and in Glasgow it is very abundant.'[83] Such sights moved a number of surgeons to exploit the opportunity which antisepsis offered.

During the early part of the nineteenth century a number of surgeons tried to operate on deformities of bone by the procedure of subcutaneous osteotomy, believing that the smallness of the

incision and use of narrow instruments would diminish the risk
of infection. This never eliminated the risk, and could not offer
an acceptable basis for a planned operation. Soon after he started
his study of the antiseptic treatment of compound fractures, Lister
showed that the antiseptic principle could be extended to the
sterilisation of hands and instruments, and carried out elective
operations on malunited fractures. By 1869, when Ogston visited
Hector Cameron in Glasgow, Cameron was exploring the knee
joint as an accepted part of his surgical work.

Then in 1872 Professor Volkmann of Halle visited Lister in
Edinburgh and was convinced of the potential of the antiseptic
system. Returning home, he introduced the full Listerian regime
into his 'old, always overcrowded hospital, which offers the most
unhygienic conditions', and over two years he successfully treated
31 compound fractures. Impressed by this test of antisepsis, he had
the confidence to follow Lister into the field of planned surgery.
During 1874 Volkmann performed 13 osteotomies on the bones of
the leg, with uneventful recovery. Lister presented a translation of
Volkmann's report in Edinburgh in December 1874.[84] Annandale
in Edinburgh then led the way in March of 1875 when he removed
a wedge from the lower end of the femur for knock-knee (fig. 5.8).
In the following month Macewen performed an osteotomy on the
shaft of the femur for ankylosis of the knee. Ogston introduced
his operation for knock-knee in May 1876, and was soon followed
by Chiene in Edinburgh, Barwell in London, and Macewen, who
began his series of osteotomies for *genu valgum* (knock-knee) in
May 1877.[85]

Ogston's operation was open to the objection that the osteotomy
on the inner condyle extended the cut into the knee joint, and so
altered the articular surfaces (although these changes did not seem
to affect most patients in the long term). Macewen's operation
left the joint intact, and obtained correction of the deformity by
cutting transversely across the shaft of the femur directly above the
condyles, stopping short of dividing the outer surface of the femur.
He then manipulated the lower leg to fracture this remaining
segment of bone and allow the lower leg to swing inwards, until it
was straight, and could be splinted until it healed (fig. 5.8).

By 1877–78 Macewen had modified his antiseptic technique. He

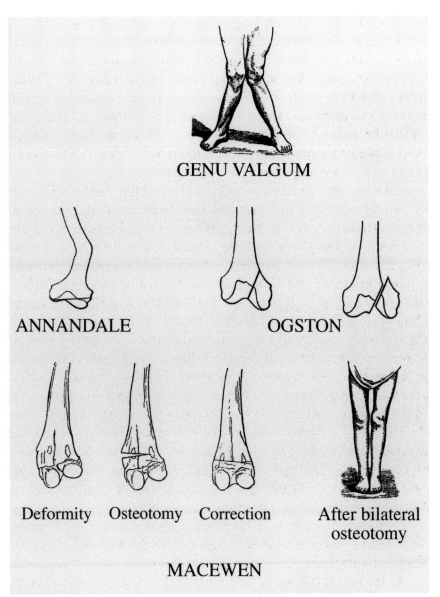

Fig. 5.8. Three operations for *genu valgum*. Annandale removed most of the articular surface of the femur, and Ogston reshaped it. Macewen improved on this by removing a wedge from the femoral shaft, thus leaving the articular surface intact. (P.F.J.)

was thoroughly washing and scrubbing arms, hands and nails, and wearing a freshly laundered gown whenever he and his assistants operated. His chisels and osteotomes were made to his own design by a Glasgow blacksmith, Mr T. H. MacDonald, who forged them from a single piece of steel. Macewen was closely involved in the minutiae of forging, aiming to obtain the greatest hardening of the cutting edge of the blade, while leaving some resilience within the blade, to avoid snapping. Any instrument with a wooden or bone handle was now discarded because dirt could lodge in any cracks. Macewen was moving towards sterilising his instruments in boiling water (as had been advised by Pasteur back in 1874). Macewen applied to the Managers for a utensil which could act as a steriliser but they were not helpful. A few days later, during a ward round, Macewen found a shining new fish kettle lying in a prominent position: no one had laid claim to it so he took it to the theatre where, over a gas ring, it served as the instrument steriliser for many years. It was Macewen's daughter Margaret who revealed its origin:[86] some twenty years later Macewen was a passenger on the Canadian Pacific Railway when the train stopped in Calgary. A local doctor approached Macewen and offered him a pressing invitation to visit a new hospital out in the country. Macewen indicated that he could hardly expect the train to wait for him, but the doctor assured him that the train would not leave without him – which became understandable when it emerged that the doctor was also the local sheriff. They drove off and at the hospital Macewen was introduced to a Sister who had trained at the Royal Infirmary in Glasgow. At a suitable moment the Sister asked to speak quietly with Macewen, and proceeded to tell him the origin of the fish kettle – the nurses of the ward knew of his fruitless request for a steriliser and decided to club together, buy a kettle, and leave it in a place where he would find it. Macewen was deeply appreciative of this news, received in strange circumstances, for he had never been able to explain the origin of the well-used kettle.

For the time being Macewen continued to rely on antiseptics for cleaning the operation site with 1-in-20 carbolic lotion, and the drapes were soaked in it: he operated under the carbolic spray. These precautions were certainly effective. Macewen performed his first osteotomy for knock-knee in May 1877, and by September 1880 he could report on 330 patients with bony deformities of the leg, of whom 220 had knock-knee, and 64 had bowed legs. A total of 835 osteotomies had been performed on 557 legs, an operating rate of about 12 patients requiring 20 osteotomies in every month. Of the 835 osteotomies – each one a deliberate creation of a compound fracture – only eight showed evidence of sepsis, which cleared up in every case.[87] By any standard this was an outstanding result for the operating technique which Macewen, following Listerian principles, had evolved. It was an equally outstanding tribute to his pre-operative assessment of the patients, the skill of the anaesthetists and the quality of the nursing care back in the wards. Children and young people who suffered from rickets were almost certain to be poorly nourished, and in a low state of health: understandably, 'in my earlier osteotomies the strong and healthy were selected'.[88] However, it soon became apparent that this rule 'excluded many patients whose limbs most needed strengthening'. As experience was gained, Macewen realised that 'with care an antiseptic osteotomy can be performed in the weak and enfeebled with impunity'. Only three patients died, one from tuberculous meningitis, one from diphtheria and one from pneumonia. Convalescence was slower in the more feeble, but then their restored mobility meant that their general health improved, as did their morale. Macewen concluded, 'The patient feels you have taken away a reproach from him, you have enabled him to earn his bread, and you have placed him on a footing of equality with his fellows.'[89]

In 1884 Macewen attended an International Medical Congress in Copenhagen, at which *genu valgum* was the topic for one session. He was able to report that the total number of patients undergoing an osteotomy for deformity had risen to 704. Of these, 490 had *genu valgum*, with 820 osteotomies being performed on 804 limbs. All had been carried out under full Listerian precautions. The number of cases of sepsis had risen to eight, and there had been two further deaths, from pulmonary tuberculosis and from diphtheria, a total of five deaths. The late results were uniformly encouraging.[90] Ogston was also in Copenhagen, and he rose to say that, after considerable experience with his own operation, he had concluded that Macewen's operation gave results superior to his own, and this was the advice he gave to his students.[91] After these generous words, many others reported good results with Macewen's operation, while others favoured Ogston's procedure. A perceptive leader in *The Lancet* summed up the situation:

> The reason why Dr Macewen and others can show an almost unbroken success in their long list of cases is that each has been the subject of special care; familiarity with the details of the operation has not been allowed to beget neglect of any necessary precaution ... The large number of cases recorded by Dr Macewen, Dr Ogston and other surgeons, has now settled the position of this operation. The safety of the procedure has been demonstrated, and it is only necessary to insist upon careful observance of all the precautions indicated by experienced operators.[92]

Within 13 years of the publication of Lister's first paper on the antiseptic principle, the practice of elective surgery had been transformed.

Here it seems appropriate to recall another story told by Macewen's daughter, Margaret.[93] After he had left Glasgow for Edinburgh, Lister paid a return visit, and he called on Macewen. They were walking from Macewen's wards at the top of the Fever Hospital, across a bridge which linked them to the Surgical Hospital. Lister said, 'Macewen, do you find this bridge a convenience?', remarking that he had persuaded the authorities to erect it. Macewen replied, 'Yes it is a convenience, but that is nothing compared to the greater gangway you provided by which patients after operation cross directly from the wards into the midst of life and health.' Macewen received a kindly look, a suppressed smile and a pressure of the arm, and then Lister said, 'Well, Macewen, if I built the bridge, you at least have made good use of it.'

CHAPTER SIX

A Decade of Movement in Antiseptic and Aseptic Surgery, 1880–1890

The latter half of the nineteenth century was a period of remarkable progress, in ways which extended well beyond any developments in surgery, and it was comprehensively initiated in the Great Exhibition of 1851. This was inspired, and to a great extent realised, by Prince Albert, Queen Victoria's consort. He was expertly rescued from planning controversies when Joseph Paxton produced detailed plans, within ten days, for a Crystal Palace – 'the blazing arch of lucid glass'[1] – which accommodated the exhibits. It celebrated the growth of industry, manufacturing and enterprise which had transformed the country since 1800. More than six million people attended before the exhibition closed.

For the first time in mainland Britain the number of people living in towns and cities exceeded those living in the countryside, so great were the demands of industry for labour. In Glasgow the local availability of raw materials promoted the manufacture of iron and steel, which in turn resulted in its skills in shipbuilding and railway engineering becoming world-famous. Dundee developed into a great processor of jute. Aberdeen was already a major textile and shipbuilding centre: the series of wooden clippers built between 1840 and 1870 to carry emigrants to Australia, and return with tea from China were unique. *Thermopylae*, built for the White Star Line in 1868, made a maiden voyage to Melbourne in 61 days, which remains an unbeaten record for a ship under sail.[2] Granite from Aberdeen had supplied London with setts and paving stones since the eighteenth century. In the

1830s Alex Macdonald devised steam-driven machinery to dress and polish the hard stone building-blocks, and soon 60 polishing yards were kept busy with large export orders, especially to the USA.[3] In 1868 the *Flying Scotsman* began its daily run between London King's Cross and Edinburgh Waverley, covering the 393 miles in ten hours.

Just ten years after the success of the Great Exhibition, when he was exerting a valuable influence on the Queen in affairs of state, Prince Albert fell seriously ill in November 1861 and on 14 December he died of typhoid fever. This was a reminder that even at Windsor the 'cesspools still made parts of the Castle almost uninhabitable'[4] – conditions which must have offered a constant risk to health. Across the country at this time 'the sanitation of the early nineteenth century did not differ materially from that of the fifteenth century'.[5]

This continued failure to see the connection between poor sewage disposal and the contamination of water supplies resulted in recurrent outbreaks of cholera. In Glasgow primitive housing conditions resulted in cholera epidemics in 1832 and 1848–49, when 4,000 deaths occurred. In London the epidemic of 1854–55 was the occasion when John Snow made the crucial observations on the water supplied by the Lambeth and the Vauxhall Water Companies, which proved that cholera was a water-borne disease.

Faced with some of the worst of these problems, Glasgow found 'the energy and public spirit to attempt the most basic solutions – summed up in the phrase "municipal socialism", although it was initiated by Liberals and Tories'.[6] The first scheme to emerge was the Glasgow Corporation Waterworks Act of 1855. This resulted in a great piece of civil engineering which brought into the city 50 million gallons of clean water each day from Loch Katrine, 35 miles to the north. When it was opened in 1859 the aqueduct ran in 13 miles of tunnelling, and was carried over 25 major rivers and valleys. As a consequence, when cholera returned to Glasgow in 1865 there were only 66 cases.[7] The other Scottish cities engineered similar aqueduct schemes in the 1860s. Aberdeen took water from the river Dee at Cairnton, 20 miles upstream from the city, while Edinburgh and Dundee obtained their water from lochs in the Borders and in Angus. It took longer for these cities to devise effective schemes for sewage disposal.

London tackled this problem from the opposite direction. When in 1858 the Queen and Prince Albert attempted a cruise on the Thames, 'its malodorous waters drove them back to land, and Parliament rose early because of the "Great Stink"'.[8] These miseries finally enforced change and in August 1858 Disraeli's bill to establish the Metropolitan Board of Works became law. The Board authorised Joseph Bazalgette to start on his remarkable scheme to prevent sewage entering the Thames in London. His plan involved the building of 165 miles of underground main sewers, with innumerable local tributaries. One main sewer ran beneath the Victoria Embankment and then under Fleet Street, and on to the collecting point far to the east. The outfall into the Thames estuary was at Barking on the north shore, and Crossness on the south.[9]

In the remaining thirty years of the century Glasgow truly embraced the notion of 'municipal socialism'. Town gas flowed through the mains, trams ran in the streets, public bathhouses were built, and libraries and an art gallery came into being.[10]

In Scotland elementary education in parish schools was introduced in the sixteenth century by John Knox and his followers. This had developed into a strong tradition, and Scottish children were generally well-grounded in the three Rs and the Protestant religion. However, the children of the large families of the poor could earn useful money, and schooling often ceased at age 8 or 9. The Education Act of 1872 made school attendance compulsory between 5 and 13, but fees were only abolished in 1891, so attendance was far from universal.[11] For those who could read, taxes on paper had been lifted and in 1863 there were more than 1,000 newspapers in Britain, mostly of recent origin.[12] In a golden age for literature, between 1850 and 1872, all the major novels of Elizabeth Gaskell, George Eliot, Charles Dickens and Anthony Trollope were published.

The education of women was making significant progress. Girton College in Cambridge opened in 1873. After a long struggle, Elizabeth Garrett became the first woman to be licensed to practise medicine in 1865, but she had to go to Paris to graduate MD in 1870. There followed the opening of the School of Medicine for Women in London in 1874. In 1856 Florence Nightingale was given a heroine's welcome when she returned from the Crimean campaign, and in 1860 she opened the Nightingale School of Nursing at St Thomas' Hospital. Its initial purpose was to train senior nurses, and some of the graduates of the school became matrons in Edinburgh (1871), Aberdeen (1878) and Glasgow (1879).[13] Over time these pioneers achieved major improvements in nursing practice and conditions.

In the wider world Abraham Lincoln became President of the USA in 1860, followed by the miseries of the Civil War. In 1870 the Franco-Prussian war established the vigour of the new Prussian state. In 1877 Queen Victoria was declared Empress of India, amid celebrations of the extraordinary extent of the British Empire. In Parliament there were the alternating reforming governments of Disraeli and Gladstone.

James Clerk Maxwell deserves to be more widely remembered. Born in Edinburgh in 1831, at the age of 25 he was appointed Professor of Natural Philosophy at Aberdeen. Eventually he became Professor of Experimental Physics at Cambridge, where he planned and inaugurated the famous Cavendish Laboratory. An outstanding mathematician, in the 1860s Maxwell found that as a fluctuating electric current flowed along a wire, it sent electromagnetic waves rippling out into space which moved at the speed of light. In the 1880s Hertz proved the existence of these waves by experiment, and then Marconi demonstrated that they could be detected across the breadth of the Atlantic. Wireless communication soon followed. Maxwell's life work covered a wide area of mathematics and physics, and it was Einstein who claimed that 'one scientific episode ended and another began with James Clerk Maxwell'.[14]

In 1859 Charles Darwin published *On the Origin of Species*, which was the product of many years of observation and cogitation. By 1872 it had run through six editions, provoked long-lasting debate and given an enduring stimulus to scientific thought and investigation. 'His method was to spin a hypothesis, and then deduce from it consequences that should follow, which could be refuted or verified.'[15] Eight years later Lister published his first papers on the antiseptic system, and provoked a similar continuing debate in the world of surgery. There is no record of a meeting between the two men, but they could certainly have shared experiences.

Lister in London

When in June 1877 the Listers learned that they would again be on the move, this time to London, Joseph had – among many other matters – to decide on a theme for his Inaugural Lecture as Professor of Clinical Surgery at King's College. It is generally forgotten that Lister had been engaged throughout the Edinburgh years in extensive research into the bacteriology of fermentation. The results were interesting and he decided to lecture on this subject, which he believed to be fundamental to an understanding of the cause of wound infection.

The Listers' Edinburgh notebooks contain full reports on these experiments, and visitors to the study at 9 Charlotte Square were likely to be shown something of the work in progress. Lister's dresser, John Leeson, writing fifty years later about his first visit to the house in 1875, remembered that Lister 'led me to a long table on which were rows of test tubes covered with glass shades, half-full of various liquids, and in the mouth of each was a plug of cotton wool. With great care and pride he picked out one here and there, held it up to the light, and seemed inexpressibly pleased at its condition – this was clear, this was turbid, and this was mouldy. I wondered what connection they could have with any branch of surgery. Though I had spent 2 years at one of London's most up-to-date hospitals I had never heard anything about microbes.'[16]

Following Pasteur's work on fermentation, Lister realised that if microscopic germs carried in the dust suspended in the air could cause sugar solutions to ferment, then it was possible for dust carrying harmful germs to gain access to living tissues, through wounds in the skin, and cause putrefaction. His subsequent success with the antiseptic treatment of compound fractures had given support to this theory: it strongly suggested that by applying carbolic acid to visibly contaminated wounds he had killed harmful germs lying within them. However, the very existence of such germs was still in the 1870s widely rejected, and Lister knew that he needed to provide objective evidence of the existence of germs causing putrefaction. If by experiment he could show that it was contamination by living germs that caused raw milk to turn sour – a form of putrefaction – this would be important evidence.

When Lister started work on this subject in the early 1870s, bacteriology as a science barely existed so, like Ogston a few years later, the Listers had to feel their way (fig. 6.1). Lister devised an iron-clad hot box in which his glassware could be sterilised at 300°F – a forerunner of the autoclave. He found that the souring of cows' milk, in which milk-sugar (lactose) is converted into lactic acid, was due to a specific germ, *Bacterium lactis*: souring never occurred unless this germ was present.[17] Souring could be delayed indefinitely by boiling the milk and then keeping it in a sterile test-tube which admitted air but prevented access to dust: there was therefore no intrinsic tendency for milk to sour (fig. 4.1, p. 80).

The Listers' particular contribution was to practice progressive dilution of a culture of *B. lactis*. In a series of laborious experiments they obtained a suspension so dilute that a single drop contained a single germ of *B. lactis*. At this dilution they found that if each of five test tubes of boiled milk were inoculated with a single drop of the suspension, only one or two tubes underwent souring. Where this did not occur the suspension was too dilute to contain even one germ. This meant that souring could only take place in the presence of a pure culture of *B. lactis* – a specific germ was producing a specific effect. This was objective evidence of the germ theory of putrefaction.[18]

There is no doubt that the Listers were unfortunate to be working in 1875–77, just before the aniline dyes were found in Germany to allow the staining of bacteria, so making them easily visible under the microscope. Ogston, who started work in the following year, was certainly helped in his more direct investigation of surgical sepsis by the publication of Koch's two books on the staining and microscopy of bacteria.

Reading the Inaugural Lecture again now, one has to wonder whether, in his enthusiasm to communicate an important piece of research, Lister failed to recognise that he was asking quite a lot

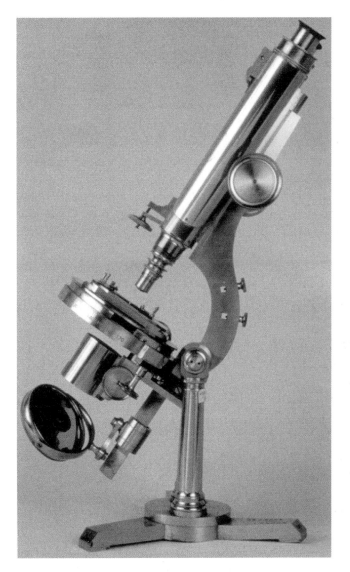

Fig. 6.1.
Lister's
microscope. It
incorporated
the achromatic
lens designed
by his father,
J. J. Lister,
which
eliminated
colour
distortion. This
instrument
was built by
Lister's cousins,
Richard and
Joseph Beck.
(Royal College
of Surgeons
of England)

of his audience. It is a closely argued thesis, with a good many sub-clauses, which would demand close attention from a mixed assembly of Fellows of the Royal Society, practising surgeons, and lively students. It was quite a step to expect instant understanding of the connection between the evidence in many tubes and flasks containing sound and sour milk, and to transfer this to the raw facts of surgical sepsis.

On 11 September 1877 Joseph and Agnes travelled from Edinburgh to London, once again nursing a collection of glassware which they had prepared for the lecture. Lister had already taken the lease on 12 Park Crescent and there, next day, he set up his specimens in the room set aside as a laboratory, checking that they had not suffered from the journey. Today the Crescent remains, unchanged outwardly, as the termination to Portland Place, the whole scheme having been designed by John Nash in the 1820s. Just across the road lay Regent's Park, where Lister could take his morning walks. The Listers then left for a holiday among the Italian Lakes, Agnes providing a most attractive description of an expedition to climb Mount Bre, near Lugano.[19] While they were away the team of assistants which Lister had assembled in Edinburgh began to arrive in London – Dr Cheyne, Dr Stewart, William Dobie and James Aitken.

The Inaugural Lecture was due to be delivered on 1 October, in the Lecture Hall of Somerset House, which was connected to the buildings of King's College in the Strand. Dr Stewart and Dr Cheyne called at the Listers' house and 'found him in his shirt sleeves, perspiring as usual, getting the exhibits in order', helped by Agnes. Then they all drove, supporting the trays and glasses as carefully as possible, to Somerset House. The audience was distinguished, but Dr Cheyne recalled 'that the majority of surgeons present could not understand what the lactic fermentation of milk had to do with surgery'. The students were bored, and responded by uttering mooing sounds whenever a cow was mentioned.[20]

For some time after Lister's arrival this lack of interest persisted among staff and students, in stark contrast to the attitude in Edinburgh. Even more troublesome was the behaviour of the nursing staff. They were Sisters of St John, a very self-sufficient nursing order, who did not recognise the teachings of Florence Nightingale, and seemed to know nothing of Lister and his work. The only patient of Lister's who was moved from his wards in Edinburgh was Lizzie Thomas, a parlour maid from Torquay, who had been admitted to the Royal Infirmary under Lister in August 1876, with a large tuberculous abscess. When Lister left Edinburgh a year later, she still required active supervision; she travelled by train in a large wicker basket, escorted by Mrs Porter, and arrived at King's College Hospital (then situated just north of the Strand) on 'a cold bleak morning at the end of October'. An extraordinary scene ensued, with the ward sister refusing to admit the patient without the consent of the Secretary, who was not due to arrive for an hour. Dr Stewart was outraged as he saw the patient getting progressively colder as she lay on the stone floor. The hall porter, a survivor of the Crimean War, was persuaded to help Dr Stewart carry Lizzie up to the ward where Stewart insisted, against all protests, that she be put to bed and made warm if not welcome.[21]

On another occasion Lister was asked to see a boy in a colleague's ward who had osteomyelitis of the femur: he was acutely ill with a high fever due to pus locked up in the marrow of the bone. He required an urgent operation, to drill the bone and release the pus. Lister went off to prepare the theatre, while Dr Stewart and the dressers returned to the ward – Edinburgh fashion – to carry the patient to the theatre. Their way was blocked by the ward sister, who demanded authority for transfer from the Hospital Secretary. Stewart pointed out that he had left and would not return until the following morning. Opposition continued, most of the dressers melted away, and Stewart had to pick up the patient and force his way out of the ward.[22]

During that first winter the four assistants acted as anaesthetists and supervisors of the theatre preparations, and they attended to all the dressings in the wards. This was necessary because a trained eye had to be kept on the wounds after operation, and poor supervision of wounds could have serious consequences. They made a point of attending Lister's thinly attended lectures, but in January 1878 Lister came to lecture and found no audience. The problem faced by the students was that if they quoted Lister's teachings in their final examinations, they faced the risk of being marked down by many examiners for offering misleading information.

Lister did not allow this atmosphere to interfere with his work, and Dobie's notebook shows that just two weeks after his arrival he performed a keynote operation, on a transverse fracture of the kneecap.[23] At that time to open a joint deliberately was generally condemned, and one eminent London surgeon said: 'when this poor fellow dies someone should proceed against that man for malpraxis'.[24] The poor fellow was a man of 40 who had been thrown over the head of his horse and had fallen on his right knee. He was brought to the hospital as a casualty, and admitted. Lister found a gap between the upper and lower fragments which could not be reduced by manipulation. On 26 October 1877, through a vertical incision, the surfaces of the fracture were found to be kept apart by fibrous tissue, which was cleared.

> The fragments were then drilled and a strong piece of silver wire passed through the holes and, the fragments being found to be exactly opposite, twisted up over the patella. The twisted ends were brought out of the wound, which was stitched up with carbolised silk. A small horse hair drain was introduced through a dependent opening. Strict antiseptic precautions were taken throughout.[25]

Eight weeks later, when bony union was secure, the silver wire was removed. At ten weeks the knee could be bent to a right angle and the patient was discharged. Two months later, the knee looked normal and the man could walk normally.

Then, just a month later, Lister made one of his rare excursions into abdominal surgery. Dobie again provided full notes. On a Sunday afternoon in November 1877 a man of 65 was admitted. He had a strangulated groin hernia, extending down into the scrotum, and had suffered severely from abdominal colic for two days, with persistent vomiting. The patient was in a 'completely collapsed condition'. The hernia was tense and irreducible and Lister proceeded to operation. He withdrew a length of black dead small bowel from the scrotum, removed it, and restored continuity of the bowel by end-to-end suture of the two healthy ends of bowel, using fine catgut sutures and an inverting stitch – a procedure which Lister had 'long thought about' but had not previously performed. 'The patient never recovered from his collapsed condition', and died a few hours later. At the post-mortem Lister tested his handiwork by running tap-water across the suture line – only at very high pressure was there one small leak.[26]

(This case is a reminder that although Lister had made a great advance in surgical care, he was really powerless to help a patient in surgical shock, due to repeated vomiting over 48 hours. This would produce a fluid deficit of 6–8 litres, and consequently a much reduced blood volume and blood pressure. In this state a man of 65 was a grave surgical risk. The modern surgeon would spend some hours over resuscitation with fluid given intravenously before considering an operation, but this technique did not become available for some thirty years after the 1870s. Even now, operation on such a patient, with intestinal resection, still carries a considerable risk.)

Other early operations included a major amputation through the hip joint, and an osteotomy for ankylosis of the knee joint, and helped towards the general acceptance of Lister's innovative methods. They were the subject of a clinical lecture in December to the class in the operating theatre: in a report published in *The Lancet* of 5 January 1878, Lister remarked how he felt that the class had a better chance there to see every detail, rather than gathered, several rows deep, around the bed in the ward. He concluded the published version of the lecture with a reference to the remarks which he had made in Edinburgh about teaching methods in London. These, 'made without any view to publication, may have done individual injustice, for which no one could be more sorry than myself.'[27]

This opened up an easier atmosphere, at least among medical colleagues, although it took a longer period of diplomacy to ease relations with the nurses of St John. Professor Wood, his colleague, came to Lister's wards, was impressed with the outcome of the amputation at the hip and invited Lister to collaborate in the removal of a large goitre. Lister superintended the antiseptic arrangements and Wood operated, successfully. They also removed an ovarian cyst, with a good outcome.

In 1879 the sixth International Medical Congress foregathered in Amsterdam. Lister's address was, in the words of the *British Medical Journal*, 'received by the whole Congress with an enthusiasm which knew no bounds. When he stepped forward to open his address (given in improvised French) the whole assembly rose to their feet, with repeated cheers and waving of hats and handkerchiefs. This continued for some minutes ... Lister stood, overwhelmed by this magnificent ovation.'[28] Although his reception at King's and in London was more restrained, Lister was making steady progress. In 1880 he was elected to the Council of the Royal College of Surgeons of England; having been a Fellow of the Royal Society of London since 1860, Lister was elected to its Council in 1881. He was also building up his private practice. He enjoyed the close personal relations this established with patients, and was also pleased to have the opportunity to study day by day every detail of the process of healing after an operation. His patients were often accommodated in a nursing home in Fitzroy Square, near to his house. At that time many operations were performed in the homes of patients, with trained nurses who came out from one of the teaching hospitals. Godlee described Lister's practice on these occasions.[29] The household provided basins containing carbolic acid lotion in two strengths – 1:20 and 1:40. His instruments and drapes were placed in the 1:20 lotion, sponges in the 1:40. Lister took off his jacket, rolled up his sleeves, and pinned a clean but not sterile huckaback towel over his waistcoat and trousers (for their protection rather than the patient!). The patient's skin was prepared with 1:20 lotion, and the drapes were placed around the site of the operation, held in place with safety pins. Hands were washed and repeatedly rinsed during the operation in 1:40 lotion. Lister used his own catgut for ligatures, and the wound was generally closed with silver wire or silkworm gut sutures.

In the 1880s Lister was anxious to provide a better gauze dressing than carbolic-soaked gauze, which tends to lose its effect from evaporation. In 1881 Koch recommended the use of corrosive sublimate (a non-volatile salt of mercury). This led Lister to an extensive search for a safe and reliable dressing. He finally settled on gauze impregnated with double cyanide of mercury and zinc, which was fixed to the gauze by a dye, mauveine, which had a characteristic light-purple colour. This was soon being produced in quantity by manufacturing chemists, and was widely used.[30]

After six years on the staff at King's, Lister had been producing results with antiseptic-based surgery which were consistently satisfactory, and which were steadily extending the range of general and orthopaedic surgery. These were being obtained in the wards and theatre of a London teaching hospital, where all could see that there were no secrets – provided it was understood that there was, throughout all stages up to complete healing of the wound, strict adherence to basic rules. It was here, especially back in the wards when dressings were done, that surgeons still did not recognise that rules had to be strictly followed. It was at this time that Knowsley Thornton, who had been one of Lister's house surgeons in Edinburgh, and who had become a colleague of Spencer Wells at the Samaritan Hospital, remarked that 'long after Lister came to London it was hard to find half-a-dozen surgeons in the metropolis who were competent to carry out the antiseptic treatment of a serious case'.[31]

There were, however, some important exceptions to these remarks on the London area in the last years of the nineteenth century. Arbuthnot Lane at Guy's Hospital, C. B. Lockwood at St Bartholomew's, and Cuthbert Wallace at St Thomas', were all pioneers of Aseptic Surgery. Lane favoured the open reduction of fractures of long bones and, using a 'no-touch' technique, he fixed them in their restored position with metal plates and screws – the forerunner of much modern fracture surgery. Wallace convinced his colleagues of the importance of aseptic techniques, and the theatres of St Thomas' Hospital were visited by many surgeons ready to study their methods. Later, in the 1914–18 war, Wallace was a strong advocate of immediate surgery for penetrating abdominal wounds, contrary to surgical tradition. Wallace proved his case, and laid the foundations for front-line surgery for the injured abdomen in the Second World War. C. B. Lockwood was the first person to lecture on bacteriology at St Bartholomew's, and he brought his experience together in an influential book entitled *Aseptic Surgery*.[32]

In the provinces Lister had a number of followers – Mitchell Banks and Bickersteth in Liverpool, Lund in Manchester and Pemberton in Birmingham – who all kept in touch and wrote warm and supportive letters to 'The Chief'. Back in Glasgow Hector Cameron had continued to show that the Listerian methods could produce consistently good results, and in 1873 he was appointed Full Surgeon in the Royal Infirmary. He was a popular teacher among the students – 'by his example he taught us veracity, concern for the best interests of the patient, care for the feelings of others, and a warm and broad humanity. As an operator he was methodical, calm and self-reliant, without showmanship, and he was remembered for his ward visits late in the day, to check on the post-operative patients.'[33] The two friends kept in close touch and in 1879, rather lonely in London, Lister wrote to Cameron saying, 'I often think of you and wish I could drop in.'[34] Lister had been very much an Englishman when he went on his first visit to Scotland in 1853. This was supposed to last for a month, but after 24 years Scotland had become his home, and, although he probably believed that his return to London was proving worthwhile, he had comparatively few friends, and never felt wholly at home.

The Transition from 'Antiseptic' to 'Aseptic' Surgery

Between 1875 and 1890 there were many surgeons, especially in Scotland and Germany, making changes to the strict Listerian regime, with its reliance on destroying germs with carbolic acid. These changes aimed at achieving sterility of instruments and dressings by the application of heat rather than chemical solutions. Lister's regime was well established and so it continued to be called the 'antiseptic' regime. To distinguish the new methods based on heat, they acquired the name of 'aseptic' operating techniques. This was unfortunate and confusing, for the aim of both regimes was to achieve the state of 'asepsis' – the absence of septic germs – on their instruments. However, the term had come to stay.

Macewen in Glasgow embraced Lister's teaching wholeheartedly, and when reporting on his hundreds of osteotomies stated that 'the operations have been conducted throughout under the spray, with strict Listerian precautions'.[35] However, he soon made modifications in his operating room at the top of the Fever Hospital – the room was thoroughly cleaned and redecorated, hands arms and fingernails were thoroughly scrubbed, and he wore a freshly laundered gown (fig. 6.2). The osteotomes were made in one piece of steel and were sterilised in boiling water in the famous fish-kettle. The use of antiseptics was restricted

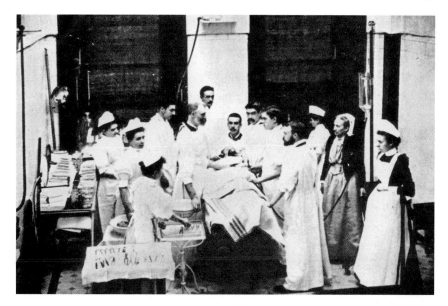

Fig. 6.2. Macewen at work in his operating theatre, in the Glasgow Royal Infirmary, in 1892. Nurses and doctors wore freshly laundered gowns, with the sleeves rolled up, and hands and arms thoroughly scrubbed. Instruments, which had been sterilised by boiling, were laid out on a dry sterile towel. (Turner, G. G., *The Macewen Outlook in Surgery*, Glasgow, 1939: 24)

to cleaning the skin of the patient with 1:20 carbolic lotion, and drapes were wrung out in it. Macewen's views on the use of antiseptic lotions were changing, and he is reported to have said in 1879 that 'germs cannot be destroyed with antiseptic substances without at the same time affecting the tissues to which they have gained access'.[36] What moved his thoughts in this direction? There can be little doubt that it was his growing interest in the possibility of performing operations within the cranial cavity. This became a reality when, in 1879, Macewen carried out two carefully planned operations which involved opening the skull and exposing the brain. For this work he needed an 'aseptic' operating technique which did not expose the brain to chemical solutions (p. 159).

However, Macewen continued to use the spray in all his bone operations until 1884, but already opinion was moving against the value of the spray. In 1879 von Bruns abandoned the spray in his famous paper 'Fort mit dem Spray', without ill-effects, although he continued to irrigate operating wounds with 2% or 5% carbolic lotion.[37] At this time Lister's own opinion was changing. He was well aware of the discomfort which the spray caused around the operating table, and in 1883 wrote 'I certainly regard it as the least important of our antiseptic arrangements.'[38] In 1887 he finally accepted that the atmosphere contains few pathogenic germs, and abandoned the spray.

In this climate of opinion it seems likely that, in entering the uncharted territory of neurological surgery Macewen would employ a largely antiseptic-free regime. Everyone scrubbed up, instruments and gauze mops were immersed in boiling water, and drapes were wrung out in 1:40 carbolic lotion: very little antiseptic would reach the wound. It was Pasteur who had led the way towards an 'aseptic' technique when, back in 1874, he said: 'had I the honour of being a surgeon I would never introduce into a human body an instrument which had not been immersed in boiling water or, better still, been flamed before operation and then cooled'. Davidsohn, working in Koch's laboratory, showed in detailed experiments that all organisms (including spores allowed to dry on instruments) were killed within five minutes by immersion in boiling water containing 1% sodium carbonate: the instruments were then placed on a dry, sterile tray.[39]

In the decade 1880–90 work was also proceeding on the sterilisation of gauze dressings and surgical towels and drapes. In 1881 Koch commented on the difficulties of penetrating folded linen, and recommended passing a current of steam at 100°C through a closed chamber. Schimmelbusch, working in Bergmann's clinic in Berlin in the late 1880s, adopted Lautenschlager's vertical steam steriliser, which delivered steam under pressure in a sealed chamber to process surgical dressings and towels[40] (an example can be seen beside the scrub-up sink in the 1892 operating amphitheatre in Aberdeen (fig. 7.5, p. 185). From this pattern there have been developed modern high-pressure autoclaves working at 130°C, with careful control of the temperature achieved at the centre of packs of surgical towels.[41]

A different approach to an 'aseptic' routine was pioneered by Neuber in Kiel from 1884 with his unique design for an operating theatre, which was the clear forerunner of modern theatres. Instead of an amphitheatre which could hold hundreds of students, there was no seating for observers, the walls were plain and washable, and the floor was of concrete so that it could be hosed down. Ward clothing and dressings were removed from a patient in an anteroom.[42] Like Macewen, Neuber dressed his team in clean linen, scrubbed up, and boiled his instruments and gauze swabs for thirty minutes. This theatre design was quite original but because it was only published in 1892, it appeared too late to influence the design of the new 1892 theatre in Aberdeen.

That Neuber's example was a good one is confirmed by a story about Lister. In his 1894 monograph on aseptic technique,[43] Schimmelbusch stated that his chief, von Bergmann, Professor of Surgery in Berlin, operated in front of 100 students, while close above his head 'were placed the dusty busts of 3 great predecessors'. Lister visited Berlin in 1890 and von Bergmann was keen to show him several patients who had undergone a mastectomy, using the 'aseptic' technique. Going to the ward, von Bergmann proudly removed the first dressing – but the wound was septic. They moved on down the row of patients but each wound proved to be infected. Lister remained silent, but perhaps he wondered whether, by ill chance, some of the dust on the busts of the ancestors had blown onto the operation wounds.[44] This experience underlines why Lister remained concerned about the 'aseptic' technique throughout his life. If the surgeon relied solely on heat to sterilise his instruments and fabrics, then the ritual had to be correct in every detail, because there would be no antiseptic present, either during or after the operation, to protect the wound. Nevertheless, by 1890 there was a move to adopt the 'aseptic' regime, particularly in Germany, and Macewen's results as a pioneer of intracranial surgery were showing what could be achieved.

In 1896 the journal *Nature* carried an article by the German surgeon Tillmans which contained a useful and reconciling interpretation of the growing adoption of the 'aseptic' operating regime – 'the technique of modern surgery is based on Lister's method, and has as its watchword "asepsis without the use of antiseptics". Antisepsis has given place to asepsis, but the latter is just as surely based on the ground first broken by Lister.'[45]

Macewen and the Surgery of the Brain

The middle of the nineteenth century was a period in which, for the first time, real progress was made in understanding the workings of the brain – an organ over which there had been infinite speculation but no hard information. In 1861 Paul Broca, the Professor of Surgical Pathology in Paris, demonstrated the brain of a man who, for twenty years before his death, had been without the power of speech. He had a softening of the third frontal convolution of the brain on the left side Here Broca was introducing the wholly new concept that a particular function could be associated with a specific area of the brain – in this instance, that speech was associated with a small area in the left frontal lobe (fig. 6.3, case 1). In 1869 Hughlings Jackson in London provided clinical and post-mortem evidence showing that lesions of specific local areas of the brain were associated with specific muscular movements. In 1873 these observations were given direct experimental confirmation by David Ferrier.

Born in Aberdeen in 1843, Ferrier attended the Grammar School and the University, where he graduated MA in 1863, with first class honours in Classics and Philosophy. He then studied medicine in Edinburgh, graduating MB in 1868. Ferrier soon moved south, and in 1871 he began his life's work as a physiologist and neurologist at King's College, London (where in 1889 he became Professor of Neuropathology).

In the course of his work he was able to show that electrical stimuli applied to specific points just in front of the central sulcus of the exposed brain (fig. 6.3) stimulated specific localised muscular movements in the limbs on the opposite side of the body. Ferrier was able, for the first time, to map out the distinct area which is known as the motor cortex of the brain. Then he went on to show that, if he injured a specific point in the motor cortex, this produced weakness or paralysis of a specific movement on a contralateral limb. These bore a striking resemblance to the effects of a localised brain injury in the human.[46]

Ferrier reported this work to the Royal Society of London in 1874, and it recognised its importance by electing Ferrier a Fellow in 1876, at the age of 33. In the same year he published a book,

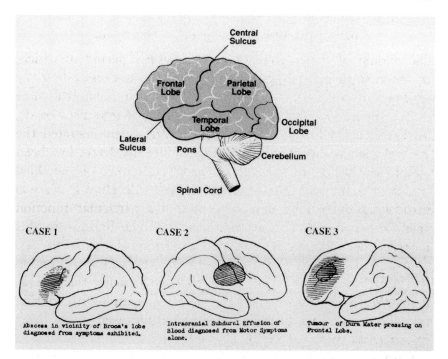

Fig. 6.3. Illustrations of the localisation of function in the cerebral cortex The uppermost figure shows the normal anatomy of the brain. The three lower figures illustrate the findings in Macewen's first three neurosurgical patients, described on pp. 159–62. (P.F.J.)

Functions of the Brain, in which he foresaw that precise analysis of an area of muscle weakness or loss of speech in a patient might lead the surgeon to explore the exact area of the brain affected by injury or disease.

Macewen knew of Ferrier's work,[47] and it chanced that he was able to apply it in the same year – 1876 – in which Ferrier's book was published. Just two months after his appointment as Full Surgeon to the Glasgow Royal Infirmary at the age of 28, a boy of 11 was admitted under Macewen's care. Two weeks previously he had fallen, striking his head above the left eyebrow, exposing the skull. By the time of admission this wound had become septic, the boy was constantly falling asleep, and his temperature was 100°F. However, when awakened he spoke sensibly, and could swallow fluids. A week later he suffered a rigor and his temperature remained high. Five days later (day 26 of the illness) he had a convulsion confined to the right arm and leg which lasted half-an-hour: he was speechless, only answering 'no, no' to every question. Macewen then made this comment:

> As it then stood, the case was clearly one of cerebral abscess, the probable site being in the third frontal convolution [that is, close to Broca's area]. Trephining and evacuating the abscess was the clear surgery [that is, a disc of bone would be removed as near to the presumed abscess as possible]. If pus sufficient to account for the symptoms were found between the skull and the dura mater, no further steps would be taken: if not the dura mater would be opened and a narrow knife would be inserted into the left third frontal convolution.[48] [Fig. 6.3, case 1]

It is necessary to pause here, and to recognise how remarkable a statement this was. Judging purely on the history and physical signs, and working on recent developments in the physiology of the nervous system, Macewen was prepared to open the skull and explore the brain, at a site away from the left frontal injury. His line of reasoning was that the rigor and high fever suggested an abscess containing pus under tension, the convulsion limited to the right arm and leg suggested pressure on the motor area anterior to the left central sulcus, while the temporary loss of speech made it likely that Broca's area was involved in the inflammatory zone around the abscess. It must be remembered that there is no evidence that, before this decision of Macewen's, any surgeon had been prepared to apply the experimental findings of the physiologists to a patient and then deliberately proceed to an exploratory craniotomy.

In the event the family did not consent to an operation, although clearly warned by Macewen of the grave outlook. On the next day the lad's temperature rose to 104°F, further convulsions followed and he died. Post-mortems were then generally accepted, and permission was given to Macewen to perform the operation, previously advised as treatment, during the autopsy. 'A disk of bone was removed from the left temporal fossa where the bone surface was congested. Between the skull and the dura there was some fluid and the dura seemed congested. An incision was therefore made in the dura mater. The brain substance was deeply congested. A narrow knife was inserted into the brain for an inch and a half, in the direction of the third frontal convolution and pus welled out.' At the end of the autopsy the skull was opened up, the whole brain removed and sectioned, revealing an abscess cavity the size of a pigeon's egg at the site of incision. Macewen commented, 'Had the operation been performed at the time it was first proposed by me, I believe the boy would have had a good chance of living and doing well.'[49] In spite of these regrets, he must have felt greatly reassured that his diagnosis had been conclusively confirmed.

Three years later three patients came under Macewen's care, each requiring intracranial surgery. The first was a boy of 9 who fell out of a window and landed on his head. There was swelling of the right side of the face and forehead and the right eye socket filled with blood. He was slightly confused. On the sixth day the left eyelids and the left side of the face began to twitch, and the boy lost consciousness for half-an-hour. Next morning he suffered convulsions, with twitching of the left side of the face, spreading to the left upper limb, and he again became unconscious. There was discolouration of the scalp in the right temporal region, where Macewen suspected there was a fracture of the skull. Macewen asked his friend Dr Robertson to see the patient, and he agreed that 'trephining was clearly indicated'. The patient was anaesthetised, Macewen made an incision in the scalp and a fracture was found 4 inches (10 cm) long. It was not depressed so a disk of bone was removed revealing a bulging dura: when it was incised 10 ml of blood and clot gushed out (fig. 6.3, case 2). Next morning the lad was 'quite intelligent', the wound healed quickly, and he made a full recovery.[50]

The second patient was a girl of 14 years, with a painful swelling in the upper margin of the left eye socket, present for some months. After several days she had three attacks of twitching of the right side of the face, spreading to the right arm and leg, with loss of consciousness. In the third attack there was marked slowing of the pulse and respiration, and the outlook became grave. Macewen decided on an emergency operation and opened the skull above the left orbit, where a tumour of the dura mater was found, compressing the left frontal lobe of the brain (fig. 6.3, case 3). This was completely removed and the wound closed. Next day the girl declared herself well, although the right-sided paralysis took some days to disappear. She went on to make a complete recovery. No microscopic examination of the tumour was made, but it is now considered to have been a meningioma (a new growth of the dura mater).[51]

The third patient had a compound depressed fracture of the skull, with considerable confusion of the intellect, and general uneasiness. The pieces of the fractured skull were considerably depressed, and Macewen decided to operate, to clean the wound and elevate the fractured pieces of bone, which had lacerated the dura. The wound healed cleanly and the patient made a complete recovery.[52]

In 1881 Macewen reported these four patients in *The Lancet* under the title – 'Intracranial Lesions, illustrating some points in connexion with the localisation of cerebral affections, and the advantages of antiseptic trephining'.[53] Professor Jefferson, a distinguished neurosurgeon writing in 1948, commented, 'The contents of this paper affirm beyond any possibility of rejection the fact that Macewen was the first to make useful application to man of the new laboratory research on the cerebral cortex. Three of the 4 cases showed unmistakably that the new brain physiology applied to man as well as to beasts, and that it could be used in the service of humanity.'[54] It must be remembered that these patients were entirely managed by careful analysis of symptoms and signs – no X-rays or other investigations were available then. Everything depended on close and continuing observation of the precise position and progression of a convulsion, so Macewen very much depended on, and paid tribute to, his nursing staff. 'In head cases it is important to have an intelligent observer in constant attendance, as the record of the first indications of the impending convulsion, and the parts affected by them, is of great use as a guide to localisation.'[55] Reading Macewen's measured words, one can feel the intensity of the responsibility he felt in embarking on these operations in wholly uncharted territory. He also notes the support he felt in 'the perfect immunity from inflammatory products which attend aseptic trephining. When the skull can be opened, the cerebral coverings incised, and the brain exposed without fear of inflammatory mischief, trephining ought to be employed, *where the localisation of the brain pressure has been established.*'[56]

During the 1880s Macewen continued to explore the surgery of the central nervous system, extending his interest to conditions causing pressure on the spinal cord. When the British Medical Association held its annual meeting in Glasgow in 1888, he was invited to speak and his address was entitled 'The Surgery of the Brain and Spinal Cord'.[57] By that time he had performed an intracranial exploration in 21 patients, when everything depended on the analysis of symptoms and signs. Eighteen of the 21 had recovered, the three patients who died being already *in extremis.* He reported a further six patients with paralysis of their legs due to pressure exerted on the spinal cord, either from acute angulation of the spinal column, or injury to it. By approaching the spinal cord from behind and removing the bony plates of the vertebrae which cover the cord he was able to relieve the pressure on the cord: this led to recovery in four of the six patients.

The first part of this 1888 paper covered the same ground as Macewen's 1881 paper. He described in detail three of the four patients there recorded and added another three similar patients cared for during 1883. During these years other surgeons had been active. In 1884, Mr Rickman Godlee (Lister's nephew), with Dr Bennett and Dr Ferrier as expert advisers, had operated in London to remove a cerebral tumour – a glioma. The patient, a young man, had died some weeks later from infection, but this was, strictly speaking, the first tumour of brain tissue to be operated on (because Macewen's patient of 1879 had a tumour restricted to the coverings of the brain – probably a meningioma). Commenting on this situation, Professor Jefferson wrote, 'However warmly we may applaud the success of the localisation in Godlee's case, it was no more than a different kind of confirmation of a physiological fact that Macewen had already proved by putting it to use.'[58] During 1886 Victor Horsley began work in London and carried out ten intracranial operations during his first year, with recovery in nine patients. When Macewen spoke in Glasgow in 1888, the full extent of his experience – from 1877 onwards – was revealed, and his paper was most warmly received. The editorial in the *British Medical Journal* commented: 'with indisputable justice may Dr Macewen claim the proud distinction of having been the leader in this country, and we believe in the world, of this great advance in our art'.[59]

At the same meeting in Glasgow, Dr Thomas Barr of the Glasgow Ear, Nose and Throat Hospital spoke of the work he had shared with Macewen on infections of the middle ear, progressing to mastoiditis. In the poor social conditions prevailing in Glasgow, chronic infections of the middle ear were common, and many quietly extended into the mastoid bone: sometimes this infection continued to spread and involved the underlying cranial cavity. Barr reported that

> we are proud to claim that ... without any swelling on the surface of the head to guide the surgeon to the seat of the abscess, but solely on the local and general symptoms and signs manifested by the patient, a collection of matter in the brain or inside the skull may be diagnosed and drained with complete success. Dr Macewen operated in 7 cases where he trephined and drained abscesses in the temporo-sphenoidal lobe of the brain, by which he has saved 5 lives.[60]

Nowadays, with antibiotic treatment of acute infections in the ear, these advanced situations are rare, but the book in which, in 1894, Macewen recorded his extensive experience, *Pyogenic Diseases of the Brain and Spinal Cord*, remains one of the classics of neurosurgical literature.[61] In it he reported on 54 patients with advanced mastoiditis and on 24 patients in whom infection had spread, necessitating an operation to drain an intracranial abscess: 23 recovered.

Jefferson rightly remarked in 1948 that surgeons today 'know more because the technical instruments for observation and exploration improve year by year, not because our mental and moral equipment increases with each generation. Improvements in operative technique are due to better lighting and ingenious electrical equipment. Let us not forget how much we owe to the path-finding men whose techniques now seem to us old-fashioned.' William Macewen is 'secure in a fame created by an internal harmony of many-sided ability and resolute firmness of character'.[62]

CHAPTER SEVEN

Consequences of a Revolution,
1890–1901

Lister gave a lecture in King's College Hospital in January 1893, when he spoke of his pleasure that, 'as the years pass, the use of the Antiseptic System has gradually spread by leavening action throughout the world'.[1]

In some cases this had happened remarkably quickly. Only months after Lister's first paper on antiseptics appeared in the spring of 1867, the news had reached a suburb of Sydney, Australia. In October of that year Dr Hogarth Pringle was using a solution of carbolic acid in glycerine to treat – successfully – an extensive compound fracture of the forearm. Because there was then no local medical journal, he reported this case in some detail in the *Sydney Morning Herald*.[2] Dr Pringle wrote warmly about his friend Joseph Lister, recalling the days when they both served Syme as his assistants in 1854. (Pringle's son, James, went on to graduate in medicine in Edinburgh. He moved west to become Macewen's house surgeon, and was for some years his assistant, before joining the staff of the Glasgow Royal Infirmary as Surgeon.)

From India reports told of how Army medical officers who followed Lister's teaching were able to transform deplorable conditions in military hospitals. Missionary doctors, many of whom had trained in Edinburgh, reported how, by keeping a stock of carbolic acid, they could soon have solutions prepared, and instruments and drapes ready for an operation.

In Germany, Austria and Switzerland Lister's work had been particularly influential, and two surgeons had built up an outstanding reputation – Billroth in Vienna and Kocher in Berne.

Billroth is remembered as a pioneer of gastric surgery. When he went to Vienna in 1867 as Professor, he set his assistants to work on animals, to devise methods of removing parts of the stomach, and then to make a safe join between the remnant of the stomach and the upper small bowel. In 1881 he was able to perform the first successful removal of a cancer of the stomach. Although Billroth did not at first accept Lister's teaching, after sending his assistants to observe his work in Edinburgh and London, he had in 1878 accepted Listerian principles, except for the spray. His 1881 patient was a woman of 43 with severe vomiting due to cancerous obstruction of the outlet of the stomach. Billroth mobilised and removed the lower half of the stomach with the adjacent duodenum, and restored continuity by joining the narrowed end of the stomach to the open end of the duodenum with fifty sutures of carbolised silk. (This is still known as the Billroth 1 operation.) At first the patient made a good recovery, but four months later she died from recurrence of the cancer. By 1890 there had been 41 operations for cancer of the stomach in Billroth's clinic, with 19 survivors.[3]

In Berne, Switzerland, Theodor Kocher became Professor of Surgery in 1872, at the age of 31, and remained at work there for the next 45 years. After graduation he spent a year travelling, visiting Billroth in Vienna, Lister in Glasgow and Spencer Wells in London. He evolved a distinctive operating technique, based on a close study of anatomy, and he was one of the first to move on from 'Listerism' to an 'aseptic' technique of sterilisation based on heat. The Swiss were particularly affected by goitres, and Kocher devoted himself to finding a safe technique of thyroidectomy, based on an initial ligation of the four arteries which supply the gland. Then, with bleeding controlled, he could work accurately on removal of gland tissue. In 1898 Kocher could report on 600 cases of thyroidectomy, with one death – a remarkable result.[4] When Berkeley Moynihan recalled his visit to Kocher he wrote:

no one who ever saw him operate in a severe case of Graves' disease [thyrotoxicosis] would ever forget his tender care, gentle touch and the deft, light, movement of every finger. Each operation was an exhibition of what perfect anatomical knowledge, a blameless aseptic conscience, the most practised technical efficiency, could accomplish. To do an operation as he thought it ought to be done, time was necessary, but there was never a moment wasted.[5]

In the United States surgeons were slow to accept Lister's work but, when they did appreciate it, proceeded to produce some outstanding surgeons. The name of William S. Halsted is still remembered as one who transformed American surgery. In 1888 he was appointed Surgeon to the new Johns Hopkins Hospital in Baltimore. In 1892 he became Professor and Surgeon in Chief, and remained in post for 30 years.[6] He is remembered for two special contributions. First, he made a major advance in the organisation of surgical training. Over the space of eight years he would take a young surgeon through a graduated system of supervised responsibility, from novice to a final two-year term as Chief Resident, when he assisted and often deputised for Halsted. These posts produced a number of individuals who, in their turn, made important advances in surgery. They were nurtured in the Halsted 'surgery of safety' – absence of haste, respect for tissues, absolute haemostasis. Second, Halsted's gentle mode of operating had great influence on surgeons. It allowed him to make meticulous dissections when operating for carcinoma of the breast, and for thyrotoxicosis, which had real effects on immediate and remote outcome.[7] Kocher, Halsted and Macewen all numbered their meticulous operations on the thyroid, and on the deformed bones of children, in their hundreds. Such numbers could only be built up in the knowledge that, by strict adherence to antiseptic/aseptic routines, safe, clean healing of their operative wounds could be anticipated.

The Mayo brothers are remembered as the founders of the Mayo Clinic in Rochester, Minnesota. The brothers William and Charles graduated in the 1880s and in 1889 opened St Mary's Hospital. There William specialised in pelvic surgery, Charles in orthopaedics, thyroid and general abdominal surgery, each brother assisting the other. This specialisation allowed them to make real advances, and by 1906 they had operated on over 300 patients with biliary tract problems, and performed a remarkable

100 gastrectomies for carcinoma. The Mayos were outstanding for studying whatever each patient could teach them, and for building up a team of surgeons who could specialise in particular areas. From these origins the Mayo Clinic arose,[8] and had a wide influence.

In Britain enterprising individuals were exploring some of the new possibilities opening up in surgery.

Harold Stiles was born in 1863 in Lincolnshire where his father and grandfather were doctors. He was apprenticed to his father at 16, and entered Edinburgh University in the following year. Stiles later wrote, 'It was a lovely evening when I first set foot in Edinburgh. Walking up Calton Hill I vowed that I would endeavour to make my home in Edinburgh, and that I would not leave unless I was starved out.'[9] When he graduated in 1885, with first-class honours, he became house surgeon to the Professor of Surgery, John Chiene, in the Royal Infirmary, and then became his assistant. Chiene had been Lister's assistant, and was his faithful disciple after Lister left Edinburgh for London. Chiene was also remarkable for creating the first pathological laboratory to be attached to a surgical ward. There, perhaps for the first time in the United Kingdom, the pathology and bacteriology of specimens from his patients were examined. Here Stiles made his home and carried out basic research on the pathology of carcinoma of the breast.

After his appointment as a junior surgeon to the Infirmary, Stiles took six months' leave to work with Kocher in Bern, and there fell under his spell. Kocher's adoption of the 'aseptic' technique of operating convinced Stiles that it was a real advance on Listerian methods, and on his return to Edinburgh he introduced the 'aseptic' regime. In 1898 Stiles followed Joseph Bell as Surgeon to the Children's Hospital, and for the next twenty years he steadily extended the range of the surgery of infancy and childhood (fig. 7.1).

Stiles' most influential work was done in the field of tuberculosis of bones and joints. It is easy now to forget how at that time this disease dominated hospital work[10] (fig. 7.2). Lister spent much of his time on this subject, both with children and adults, and Stiles followed him in the careful surgery which conserved limbs

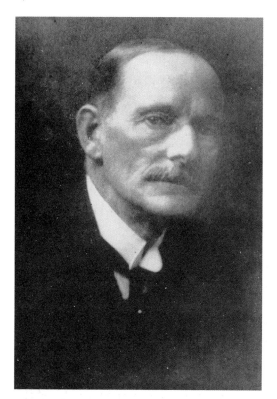

Fig 7.1. Harold Stiles. One of the first surgeons in the United Kingdom to devote himself, for over 20 years, to the surgery of infancy and childhood. (Brown, J. M. M., *Journal of the Royal College of Surgeons of Edinburgh* 1956, 1: 316–18)

Fig. 7.2. Chart showing admissions to the Hospital for Sick Children in Edinburgh, 1897–1941, for Tuberculosis of Bones and Joints, Abdominal Organs, and lymph glands in the neck. (Robarts, *Journal of the Royal College of Surgeons of Edinburgh* 1969, 14: 299–315)

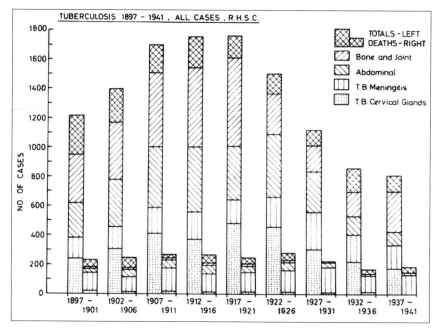

by excising affected joints, rather than resorting to amputation. Between 1901 and 1910 he performed 200 excisions of joints in the limbs of children. Equally important, he set his assistant, John Fraser, to work on the basic pathology, especially on the role of the bovine form of tuberculosis. After much painstaking work, Fraser showed that tuberculosis of bones and joints, and of the lymph nodes in the neck (scrofula), was due in 60% of cases to infection from milk. Part of Fraser's research was a field study in the north of Scotland that revealed the high incidence of tuberculous disease of the udder among cows. This led on to a vigorous campaign to examine milk supplies, and to promote the pasteurisation of milk, which had been introduced in the 1880s.[11]

Another interest of Stiles was in the causes of incontinence of urine in childhood. He took up one particularly distressing condition, epispadias, in which a girl is born with an open bladder neck, which means that she has no control over the flow of urine. As the first year passes it becomes clear to the parents that their child is constantly wet, and this shows no sign of improvement. Although these children are otherwise healthy, one of Stiles's patients aged 7 was 'of a very timid and emotional disposition, due it is said to the father having taken an antipathy to the child on account of her disability. There were 5 other children in the family, all healthy.'[12]

Stiles could find no record in the literature of a reliable method of securing continence. It was clear to him that no local operation on the bladder neck would be fully effective. He concentrated on the idea of transplanting both ureters, to drain into the upper end of the rectum. Urine would then accumulate in the continent rectum, and could be released at will through a normally functioning anal canal. Attempts at doing this had, however, produced very poor results. Stiles devised an operation which allowed each ureter to be disconnected from the bladder and then made to pass obliquely through the rectal wall. This oblique track acted as a valve, so preventing reflux from the septic rectum, up the ureter, to the kidney. Three years after he had performed this operation on two girls, he was able to report to the American Surgical Association that they had remained in good health, able to run about freely and play games.[13] They were completely dry by day, and there was only an occasional leak at night. This has remained a standard method ever since. Stiles had the pleasure of meeting one of his old patients at a surgical meeting in Edinburgh some 23 years after her operation: she had remained dry and well ever since.

Stiles remained a very active children's surgeon until 1919 when he was recalled to the Royal Infirmary to be Regius Clinical Professor of Surgery. He became a renowned teacher in the lecture room and operating theatre. Then, one day in 1925, at the age of 62, he finished his out patient clinic, said goodbye to his staff, and retired, without fuss or any further participation in medical matters. He devoted himself to botany and geology. There was much speculation over this sudden move. His close colleague, John Fraser, commented, 'There were days when he was conscious of being very weary: as he could not bear the thought of a gradual decline, he felt it preferable to lay down his task while his powers were still unspoiled.'[14]

Lawson Tait was to make a major contribution to the development of abdominal surgery. Born in 1845, he matriculated at Edinburgh University in 1859, and in 1862, at the age of 17, he was attending Syme's lectures, and lodging in James Simpson's house. He always honoured Syme for his operative skill and wise judgment, and Tait later remembered how 'Syme was always perfectly dressed, and as clean as a new pin. From his boots to the top of his head, no one ever saw dirt, disorder or the appearance of hurry. He was always washing his hands – I think I may say he washed them every time he touched a patient, and his assistants had to be like him.'[15]

Qualifying in Edinburgh in 1866, at the age of 21, Tait first worked in Wakefield. There, by 1870, he had already performed three ovariotomies, and had been awarded the Fellowship of the Edinburgh College of Surgeons. In the following year Tait moved to Birmingham, and joined the staff of the Women's Hospital as Junior Surgeon. He could never accept that germs caused surgical sepsis, but when he looked at the results of his first fifty ovariotomies he found that his mortality rate was 38% – at a time when Wells and Keith were reporting much lower rates. Tait had to think again. He never accepted Lister's methods but, remembering

Syme's principles, he resolved to follow his rule of cleanliness. Tait evolved a technique in which he worked in a small hospital, with a trained nursing staff. He made free use of soap and water, while instruments and ligatures of silk thread were sterilised in boiling water. Tait was careful about the use of sponges – which were difficult to sterilise – and preferred to use a sucker to keep the operation field clear of blood. He liked to wash out the abdomen with boiled water. This technique comes close to the 'aseptic' regime and, gaining confidence, he decided to abandon the clamp on the abdominal wall in ovariotomy. Tait adopted ligation of the stalk of the cyst with sterile silk, cut the ligature short, dropped the pedicle back and closed the abdomen. By 1882 Tait had reduced his mortality to 3%, and in 1886 he reported 136 consecutive ovariotomies without a death[16] (fig. 7.3).

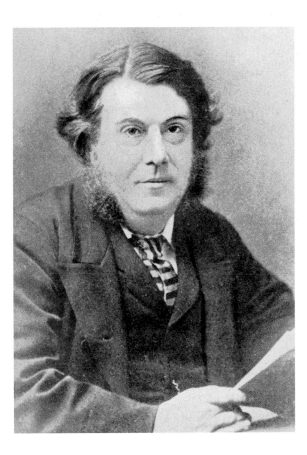

Fig. 7.3.
Lawson Tait in 1891, aged 45. This photograph was taken at the peak of his career, only eight years before his death. (McKay, W. S., *Lawson Tait*, London, 1922)

These results gave Tait the confidence to explore further opportunities in the surgery of the abdomen. He started to remove large chronic abscesses involving the ovary, which were a common but poorly treated source of chronic lower abdominal pain, with promising results. It is also now clear that Tait was the first British surgeon to remove an acutely inflamed appendix, in 1880.[17]

A girl of 17 complained of pain in her right groin, which had grown worse over several weeks. Finding a swelling above the groin, with a crackly feel, a fever of 39°C and a pulse rate of 140 per minute, Tait incised a large abscess extending down into the pelvis, and there came upon a black, gangrenous appendix, which he removed. He placed a drainage tube deep in the pelvis and closed the incision. The girl made a complete recovery.

It is clear that Tait cannot be said to have made a pre-operative diagnosis of appendix abscess: what he did was to diagnose an acute abdominal abscess which – like acute abscesses elsewhere in the body – needed surgical drainage. He felt that he had sufficient experience in the abdomen, and proceeded to explore it. At that time acute appendicitis was barely recognised, and these cases were named 'acute typhlitis', because they were thought to be due to inflammation in the caecum. Recognition of acute appendicitis still lay some years in the future.

There were no aids to diagnosis in the abdomen at that time – just the five senses had to be exercised at the bedside – and understandably this inhibited an active surgical approach to abdominal disease. It was Tait's particular contribution to argue that 'it is right to open the abdomen where there is evidence of disease which is threatening life, or making it a burden'.[18] A diagnosis could then be made and appropriate treatment carried out.

This led Tait to explore the upper abdomen, an area which had scarcely been touched so far, because diagnosis was more difficult. The ovaries and uterus often produced swellings which had specific signs, which could be interpreted by careful examination, but in the upper abdomen there was a greater variety of organs; they were more inaccessible, and produced a greater variety of symptoms and signs.

In 1879 Tait saw a woman of 40 who had suffered pain in the right upper abdomen for a year, and a mobile mass could be felt there. Tait consulted his colleagues, whose opinions varied, so he decided to explore the swelling. It proved to be a distended gall bladder. It contained a large stone, which he lifted out, and another was impacted in the neck of the bladder: this he broke up. Tait sutured the opening in the gall bladder into the incision and the patient made a good recovery. At the time it was not recognised in Britain that Bobbs in Indianapolis and Kocher in Bern had performed a similar cholecystostomy, but it was Tait who went on to establish the value of the operation – five years later he reported on 14 patients, 13 of whom had recovered.[19] One of Tait's trainees – Mayo Robson – moved to Leeds and there he went on to overcome many of the problems of operating on the gall bladder and biliary passages.

There was another area in which Tait's willingness to explore the doubtful abdomen made him a pioneer, and this became his major contribution to emergency abdominal surgery. This was the arrest of acute haemorrhage from rupture of a tubal, or ectopic, pregnancy. This arises when the father's sperm progresses beyond the uterus and fertilises the maternal ovum in the Fallopian tube or oviduct. The fertilised egg then embeds in the tube, rather than in the safety of the thick-walled uterus. Between the sixth and twelfth week of foetal life the embryo and its vascular coverings have produced a significant swelling within the thin-walled tube, which readily ruptures: this involves a tearing of the developing placenta, and considerable bleeding ensues. This can be sufficient to produce serious surgical shock, with collapse of the circulation. J. S. Parry of Philadelphia had given a full account of the condition in 1876, and speculated about an operation to save the mother's life, but no one had succeeded in this.

In 1881 Tait was asked to see a woman who had been taken off the London train in a collapsed state.[20] Tait suspected that the patient had a ruptured tubal pregnancy but did not dare to operate. At the post-mortem he realised that it was technically feasible to ligate and remove the affected tube, and that it was probable that the mother's life would have been saved if he had intervened. 'After that terrible lesson I did not see another example of ruptured tubal pregnancy until I was called to Wolverhampton in January 1883. The patient was clearly dying of haemorrhage and

I advised an immediate operation.' Tait was faced with masses of clot, 'and copious bleeding at every point'. By the time Tait had stopped the bleeding the patient was at death's door. Tait realised that his approach had been at fault – he must 'make at once for the source of the bleeding, and tie the broad ligament at its base, and then remove the tube and all the clots at leisure.'[21] Two months later Tait had performed his first successful operation.

In 1888 Tait described a typical patient.[22] One evening he received a telegram from a doctor in Halifax, which said 'come at once'. The patient was aged 29, and already had four children. She had missed one period, and had suddenly collapsed five days earlier, complaining of abdominal pain and vomiting. She revived, but the pain returned, so she was kept in bed by her doctor, who suspected an ectopic pregnancy. Then, earlier that day, the patient felt sick and faint, the abdomen became distended and painful, and Tait was summoned. He found a pale, cold woman with a fast pulse, and immediately decided on operation. There was much clot and blood in the abdomen, and he went directly down to the ruptured left tube, ligated its blood supply and removed it. With the bleeding stopped he could take time over cleaning the abdomen and washing it out with boiled water. Ten days later the patient was well and up and about.[23]

This patient's history is taken from Tait's 1888 monograph on ectopic pregnancy, in which he reported 42 personal cases of acute tubal rupture with two deaths. For its time this was a remarkable record, the product of sound judgment, good timing and expert surgery.

Tait was rather too sure that his opinion was the only sensible one to hold. However, like many pioneers, this had given him the confidence to acquire exceptional experience in abdominal surgery: by the time that he retired he had performed some 5,000 operations in the abdomen. This provided a strong basis for him to establish two principles. First, it is right and safe to perform an elective laparotomy when, after proper thought, there is still a diagnostic problem (this had, in particular, allowed him to make progress in the surgery of the gall bladder). Second, in the field of emergency abdominal surgery, especially in the presence of peritonitis or haemorrhage, the surgeon should be ready to act, to catch the brief period in which the cause is still amenable to a surgical solution.

Tait was a prominent member of a team of surgeons who, in the last twenty years of the nineteenth century created the conditions which established emergency abdominal surgery as an exciting and vital element in surgical practice.

The Advent of Emergency Abdominal Surgery

This is well illustrated by the emergence of acute appendicitis as a clinical entity. Acute inflammation in the right lower abdomen was labelled acute typhlitis, and because nobody was prepared to operate, this concept lingered on. Then in 1867 Willard Parker in New York reported that it was the vermiform appendix – attached to the caecum – which could become inflamed and gangrenous: he quoted four patients for whom he had successfully drained an abscess which contained a perforated gangrenous appendix. Thereafter, 'For 20 years the Parker operation dominated the treatment of right iliac abscess in North America.'[24] It was during this period, in 1880, that Tait operated on his first case.

This period ended when the crucial paper, providing a real understanding of acute appendicitis, appeared in 1886 with the title 'Perforating inflammation of the vermiform appendix: with special reference to early diagnosis and treatment'.[25] Here Reginald Fitz, Professor of Pathology at Harvard, correlated the clinical history and post-mortem findings in no fewer than 257 patients. He concluded that 'the vital importance of the early recognition of perforated appendicitis is unmistakable. Its diagnosis in most cases is comparatively easy. Its treatment by laparotomy is generally indispensable.' Rarely can such clear advice have been given to surgeons by a pathologist.

This advice was taken up in the following year by T. G. Morton in Philadelphia, who made a pre-operative diagnosis of acute appendicitis, followed by successful urgent appendicectomy. He was followed by Charles McBurney in New York, whose work is still well known to surgeons. On the basis of his first 11 patients he described what he believed to be a typical case, and published this paper in 1889.[26]

At this time American journals were not widely read in Britain, and surgeons were consequently unaware of Fitz's uncompromising advice. This slow recognition is well illustrated in the experience of the Children's Hospital in Edinburgh (fig. 7.4). One of the first to report a case in Britain was Berkeley Moynihan who, in 1895, had just been appointed Surgeon to the Leeds General Infirmary.[27] This was his first published paper, the forerunner of a large series of pioneering publications on abdominal surgery.

When Moynihan was a resident in the Infirmary he had seen a number of patients with perforated appendicitis who only arrived in the hospital when their spreading peritonitis had progressed to a stage beyond any hope of rescue. He was determined to change this situation. One of his first patients was a boy of 14 who was admitted with a two-day history of abdominal pain and diarrhoea. At 48 hours the abdomen suddenly became acutely distended, the pulse became feeble and rapid, his extremities cold and blue. The abdomen was generally tender, especially over the right lower quadrant. Moynihan diagnosed a general peritonitis, probably due to rupture of an abscess around an inflamed appendix. He opened the abdomen, drained much offensive pus, broke down loculi containing more pus, and thoroughly washed out the abdominal cavity with boiled water. He then opened, through a separate incision, an abscess above the right groin which had gangrenous walls, but he could not find the appendix. Moynihan inserted glass and rubber tube drains, closed the abdomen, and was surprised to observe how quickly the boy's condition improved. For some reason he was kept in bed for nine weeks, but he made a complete recovery. (This case, almost certainly due to a perforated appendix, would still be a worrying one today, in spite of the help which antibiotics and intravenous fluid support can give.)

Moynihan, in his commentary, was at pains to emphasise how much better it would have been to have watched this lad closely, and to operate as soon as it became clear that the signs were not improving:

> In every variety of surgical abdominal disease of an acute nature, early operative interference has a rapidly increasing number of adherents. Operation when carried out early is

practically without risk. American surgeons follow this practice and their results are, beyond all comparison, better than our own.[28]

Riddell in Aberdeen was in full agreement with this view, and in 1899 he spoke from his own experience, saying, 'no case of acute perforative appendicitis, if left to nature, recovers, but with operation the patient has a chance'.[29] However, when this paper was discussed, only a minority of the audience shared Riddell's sense of urgency. This was to be changed by a national event.

In January 1901 Queen Victoria died. She was succeeded by her son the Prince of Wales, who was due to be crowned Edward VII in June. In the middle of June he was at Windsor when he began to complain of abdominal pain and fever, and his doctor found tenderness in the right lower abdomen. On 18 June Frederick Treves, Surgeon to the King and a consultant at the London Hospital, travelled to Windsor by train, confirmed those findings, and decided to await events. Over the next two days the King's fever settled, and he felt a little better. He was determined that the Coronation should proceed, so on 23 June he travelled to London by train, and then rode on horseback from Paddington to Buckingham Palace, accompanied by a cavalry escort.[30] When Treves saw the King in the evening he strongly urged the King to consent to an operation to drain an appendix abscess, but the King was still determined on the Coronation. Treves felt the need of some support and Lister, who was also Surgeon to the King, was asked for his opinion. He agreed that drainage was needed. The King remained obdurate, so the King's Physician had to explain to him that if nothing was done His Majesty was more likely to be attending his own funeral, rather than his coronation: thereupon the King consented. On 24 June a room was prepared in the Palace by a theatre sister from the London Hospital. At 12.20 p.m. the King walked in, clad in an old dressing gown, lay down, and was anaesthetised by Dr F. Hewitt. This proved difficult the King stopped breathing twice, threw his arms about, and went black. Treves took off his jacket, rolled up his sleeves, donned an apron and scrubbed up. He made an incision over the abscess and had to go down through 4 inches (10 cm) of abdominal wall before draining a large abscess. Two rubber drainage tubes were inserted.[31]

The King made a good recovery, closely supervised by Treves: he had taken up residence in the Palace, to make sure that the abscess cavity healed from the bottom, and no loculi of pus remained undrained. In mid-July the King left for convalescence on the Royal Yacht, and his delayed Coronation took place on 9 August. He was fortunate that the slow progress of his disease had allowed adhesions to form around the inflamed appendix, so that when it perforated it caused only a local abscess, and the general peritoneal cavity remained intact. The risks were quite high, with the hospital mortality at that time standing at 26%.

This episode gave great publicity to the existence of acute appendicitis, and immediately surgical treatment became more acceptable. As earlier diagnosis and operation became more common, the mortality rate was to fall to 4–5% by 1912 (fig. 7.4). Throughout the first half of the twentieth century patients with acute appendicitis were a feature of every surgical ward receiving day, but since then the incidence of this disease has fallen steadily. A neglected case is still a dangerous condition, but with improvements in treatment a fatal outcome has become a rarity.[32]

A sharp fall in incidence has also been seen in another surgical emergency – perforation of peptic ulcers of the stomach and duodenum – which became a progressively more common condition at the end of the nineteenth century, and was a prominent feature of emergency surgery throughout the first half of the twentieth century.

Kriege, a medical practitioner in the German town now called Wuppertal, was the first to describe a successful case in 1892.[33] The patient was a man of 41 with a history of indigestion. He had been awakened by sudden abdominal pain, and when Kriege saw him at 04.00 he suspected a burst ulcer. He summoned the surgeon Heusner from a neighbouring town by telegram, but Heusner was unable to arrive until the late afternoon. Kriege had everything ready in the house for an operation; it eventually commenced at 18.30 and lasted until 21.00. A midline incision was made, offensive gas escaped, and stomach contents were seen

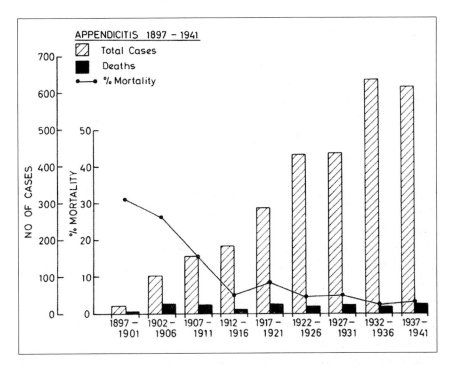

Fig. 7.4. Chart showing admissions to the Children's Hospital in Edinburgh, 1897–1941, for acute appendicitis. In the first decade of the century mortality was high (15–30%), probably due to late recognition, with consequent peritonitis. The rise in incidence continued through the first half of the century. (Robarts, *Journal of the Royal College of Surgeons of Edinburgh* 1969, 14: 299–315)

to cover the stomach and intestines. Conditions must have been most difficult as Heusner searched for a perforation, assisted by the light of a candle. Eventually, after extending the incision, he found a hole high in the stomach wall the size of a pea. He had to take large bites of the stomach wall to close the perforation. He mopped out as much of the spilt juices as he could with sterile gauze, placed some drains, and took some time over closing the incision with strong silk. The patient recovered after a long convalescence, during which a collection of pus in the chest (an empyema) was drained.

Morse, a surgeon in Norwich, was the first in Britain to report on a girl of 20 who had a perforation, also high on the wall of the stomach, which was successfully sutured.[34] She was typical of many of the patients who presented at this time – young women in their late teens or early twenties, who suffered from a curiously specific condition. They were unmarried and most were employed as housemaids: in case after case the perforation was high up on the stomach. This strange outbreak has never been explained, and it soon gave way to an epidemic of ulceration of the duodenum, in which men outnumbered women by 10 to 1. Over the first half of the twentieth century, duodenal ulceration, with its complications of perforation and sudden haemorrhage, was a feature of emergency medicine and surgery throughout Europe and North America. When Moynihan surveyed the literature in 1901, he found reports of 51 patients with a perforated duodenal ulcer: only five of them were women.[35] Mortality then was high, with only eight of the 51 surviving, mainly due to delay in diagnosis. Perforated duodenal ulcers seemed to be especially common in Scotland, and were the subject of close study in Glasgow: by the 1960s mortality had fallen to 2–3%.

Another problem in emergency abdominal surgery is presented by the patient with an obstruction of the bowels. Henry Clark, Surgeon to the Glasgow Royal Infirmary, gave an early account of such a case in 1883.[36] A miner, aged 32, was admitted to a medical ward complaining of the sudden onset, 7 days previously, of severe abdominal pain and complete stoppage of the bowels. The pulse was good and the temperature normal. 'The abdomen was much distended, tense and tympanitic, but not tender.' There was no result to an enema. Mr Clark was asked to see the patient on the ninth day of the illness, and he advised colo-puncture of the distended intestines, which yielded 'a large quantity of fetid gas, and gave much relief to the patient'. Colo-puncture was repeated, with relief, four times, but enemas were not productive. At no time did the patient vomit, and he took fluids, but he was becoming anxious and emaciated. Eighteen days after admission, and 25 days after the onset of pain, in a consultation between two physicians and two surgeons, Clark reported that they 'decided to perform abdominal section ... except the obstruction was speedily removed, the patient must slowly sink'.

The anaesthetic was given by Clark's house surgeon, using a mixture of ether and chloroform, and the abdomen was opened through a midline incision 8 inches (20cm). long. Enormously distended bowel was exteriorised and followed down to a constriction in the upper rectum, due to a torsion of the bowel. By untwisting the sigmoid colon, just above the rectum, through 3½ turns the narrowing was relieved and the bowel appeared healthy, but the large amount of gas and faeces above that point could not be evacuated. Finally, a large rectal tube was passed through the anal canal and up the rectum: six voluminous saline washouts were required before the colon was reasonably deflated. Throughout the operation the colon was kept covered with some three dozen towels dipped in hot 1:60 carbolic lotions. The abdomen was closed in layers, using chromic catgut. Although the operation lasted two hours, the pulse and respirations were easy throughout. Clark remarked, 'I was most ably assisted by Dr Macewen'. The patient made a steady recovery: diarrhoea was copious for some days but he left hospital well after five weeks. As a pioneer of surgery in intestinal obstruction, Clark affirmed: 'Abdominal section, though more risky, ensured that we should truly ascertain what we had to deal with ... it is we fear too much the custom to wait till the patient is moribund, and then very wisely decide that he is too far gone for operation.'[37] Even so, the strain of being one of the first to put this advice into effect must have been considerable.

In the following year Frederick Treves wrote a prize essay in which he gave a clear account of the ways in which the gut can be obstructed – this may be due to pressure from outside, e.g. when it is kinked in a hernial sac, from conditions in the wall, e.g. a carcinoma of the bowel, or the obstruction may lie within the bowel, e.g. impacted food. Treves, like Clark, advised his colleagues to be more ready to operate, and provided a logical basis on which to work.[38]

Lister and his Scottish Friends in the 1890s

Both Ogston and Macewen moved on to become Regius Professors, Ogston in Aberdeen in 1882 and Macewen in Glasgow in 1892. In 1882 the volume of surgery performed in Aberdeen was still remarkably low – just 200 operations in the year – but by

1888 the total had risen to 536, with 350 of these performed by the Professor. These included bone and joint operations, ten ovariotomies and a hysterectomy.[39]

This increase reflected the speedy growth in the size of the population of Aberdeen, as its industries grew. From a town of 12,000 citizens in 1801, the population had grown to 63,000 by 1841, and this had nearly doubled by 1861. The single Simpson building of the Infirmary became seriously overcrowded, and in 1887 plans were prepared for a new surgical block. This opened in 1892, with six wards on three floors, connected to two operating amphitheatres in the basement by a hydraulic lift.[40] These improved on the old theatre by having an anaesthetic room, scrub-up sinks, and electric lighting powered by a generator in the boiler house. (Even so, operating at night cannot have been easy in the light from three naked bulbs suspended over the wooden operating table.) By 1897, beside the door of the large theatre, there stood a vertical autoclave for dressings, gowns and towels, purchased from Germany for £16 5s. 0d[41] (fig. 7.5).

In 1898 Ogston completed thirty years as Surgeon to the Infirmary, and he stepped down, although he continued his teaching as Professor until he retired in 1909. The students valued Ogston's clear and memorable lectures, and at the bedside he was always mindful of the feelings of his patients. He had remained a faithful disciple of Lister and felt, justifiably, that the full antiseptic operative technique which he demonstrated to his students was one which they could safely use in any Highland castle or croft.

By 1907 the volume of surgery had doubled, from 932 operations in 1898 to 1972 in 1907.[42] By then the defects of the 1892 amphitheatre had become plain. The surgeons reported to the Board that the lighting and ventilation were inadequate, equipment was neither sufficient nor modern, and operating lists had become very long – there were only two theatres, and the large one could not be used in the morning until the surgery lecture had been delivered there – 'a most undesirable state of affairs'.[43] By this time 270 bone and joint operations, and a total of 570 abdominal operations, were being performed annually, which included major procedures on the stomach and intestines,

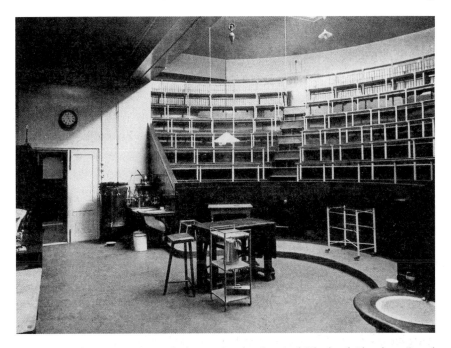

Fig. 7.5. The operating amphitheatre in the Surgical Block of Aberdeen Royal Infirmary, opened in 1892. (Levack, I. D. and Dudley, H. A. F., *Aberdeen Royal Infirmary*, London, 1992: 95)

biliary and urinary tracts, and the pelvic organs. Six ectopic pregnancies had been successfully treated. The Board decided that a vertical stack of three modern theatres, designed on the principles of Neuber, should be built, each connected to a pair of surgical wards. These were opened in 1912. (The cost was defrayed by Lord Mountstephen, who was a native of Dufftown. As a lad he had herded sheep, and then was apprenticed to a draper in Union Street, Aberdeen. He then emigrated to Canada and eventually became the Chairman of the Canadian Pacific Railway Company.[44]) The continued expansion of operative work in Aberdeen is illustrated in fig. 7.6.

Ogston had a continuing deep concern about the medical services of the British Armed Forces. After visiting medical units in France, Germany and Russia in the 1880s, he had serious doubts about the state of the medical services of the Armed Forces in Britain. He made a critical report in 1899. Then the Boer War broke out and

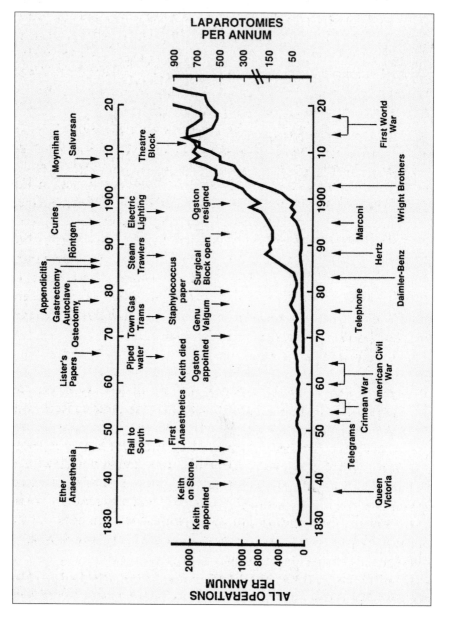

Fig. 76.
Chart of events in and around Aberdeen Royal Infirmary, 1830–1920. The legends on the top line name some events in surgery generally; on the second line social changes in Aberdeen; and on the third line, surgical developments in the City. The graph from 1830 shows annual numbers for all operations, that from 1867 gives the number of laparotomies performed each year. (Figures from Annual Reports of the Infirmary)

in June 1900, with the blessing of Queen Victoria, he visited South Africa. There he found that casualties in the British Army due to illness far outnumbered battle casualties. Thousands of the troops contracted typhoid fever but received only basic care, lying in tents on the bare ground during cold nights, with no proper nursing care. Casualties from the battlefield travelled in great discomfort in ox carts, and the standard of surgery they received was poor. Ogston himself then succumbed to typhoid and came very close to death. He paid warm tribute to the few overworked British nursing sisters, but felt very critical of senior army medical officers.[45] When he returned home he joined an expert team which made strong but constructive comments on Army Medicine.

Like Macewen, Ogston was not an easy colleague, although his patients, students and junior colleagues appreciated his high standards, humanity and sense of humour. His family knew a loving and strongly supportive father. At the age of 72, in the First World War in August 1916, he joined the British Ambulance Unit in the Italian Alps, where he was the only surgeon to serve with the Second Italian Army fighting the Austrian forces. For fifteen months he operated, often under fire and in bitter winter conditions, tending shell and grenade wounds, and cases of frostbite and trench foot.[46] This cannot have helped the severe rheumatism which clouded the rest of his life, and must have tried his lively spirit quite sorely until he died in 1929.

In 1892 Macewen became Regius Professor of Surgery in the University of Glasgow. This meant that he had to move to the new Western Infirmary, which had been built next to the new campus of the University at Gilmorehill. There was some difficulty with the managers over his accommodation, Macewen being particularly doubtful about the only operating theatre. This doubled as a student lecture theatre, and was used for social functions. For some years Macewen insisted on operating in the theatre he improvised in the corridor beside his wards, until a three-tier theatre block was built (fig. 7.7).

With his elevation to the Regius Chair Macewen resolved that his students would have the first call on his time. Two of his male

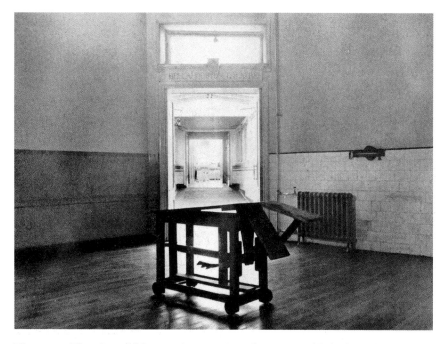

Fig. 7.7. The site of Macewen's operating theatre, established in the corridor outside his wards in the Western Infirmary. The scrub-up sinks which were installed along the walls have been taken down. (Turner, G. G., *The Macewen Outlook in Surgery*, Glasgow, 1939)

wards opened onto a large hall and here, each morning, he would seat himself on a high white stool and meet as many as 90 students. Three clerks sat alongside him, and would report their findings on one of the patients, who was brought in on a trolley. Macewen's purpose was to encourage his students to take a full history, to observe signs accurately, and then support their findings in a reasoned discussion. He looked for a thoughtful discussion rather that a quick but poorly supported diagnosis.[47]

Macewen was tall and erect, with a keen eye, and must have been an impressive figure, but he was patient, and encouraging to inexperienced but interested students. The clinic was often interrupted as he told of curious or amusing incidents culled from his experience. Then he would stride up the path to a university lecture room at Gilmorehill (fig. 7.8), and there speak of the basic principles of surgery. His operative work followed the pattern

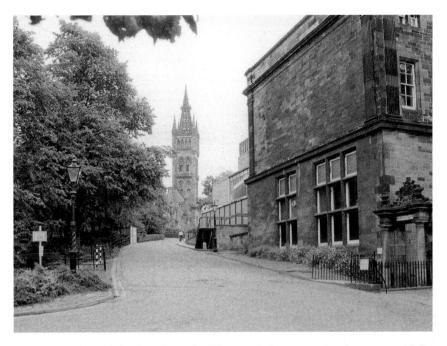

Fig. 7.8. The path leading from the Western Infirmary up to the campus of the University of Glasgow, on Gilmorehill. (P.F.J.)

which had been established at the Royal Infirmary, but the volume of work was reduced. There was, however, one remarkable addition to the fields in which he worked.

One morning in 1895, in the hospital corridor, Macewen met the Professor of Medicine, W. T. Gairdner, who invited him to a consultation. In Gairdner's ward was a young man with tuberculosis involving both lungs, complicated by a left-sided empyema (a collection of pus in the chest cavity). The man was desperately ill and breathless, with a bulging left chest that was completely dull to percussion. The heart sounds were displaced into the right chest. The patient had a fast, thready pulse and was febrile. It was clear to Macewen that the patient must soon die if left untreated: an operation was risky, but it was the man's only hope.[48]

He removed sections of two of the lower left ribs and about five litres of pus rushed out (later found to be full of tubercle bacilli, staphylococci and streptococci). It became clear that this was in fact a very large left-lung abscess. The remains of the left lung were carefully removed, and the chest cavity washed out and drained. This gave immediate relief, and the patient steadily improved. One month later Macewen carried out a left thoracoplasty (the removal of sections of a number of ribs to allow the left chest to collapse down). The remaining cavity was kept packed with gauze while it was replaced by fibrous tissue, and finally healed. The signs of tubercular disease in the right lung became quiescent, and finally the patient returned to his work as a commercial traveller.

Much later, Macewen would tell the sequel to this story. In November 1914 – some 19 years later – Macewen was out visiting a patient on a dismal foggy evening, with thin snow falling. Under a lamp on a street corner a small group of the Salvation Army stood around while one of them spoke. Macewen paused, realised that the speaker was the man with one lung, and that he was speaking of his Saviour. Their eyes met, the speaker hesitated, stopped and, eyes downcast, said – 'Amen'.[49]

It was often said that Macewen was so much an individualist and innovator that he had to do everything for himself, leaving little operating to his assistants. One reason for this was noted by Duguid, his house surgeon. He pointed out that Macewen's university lecturers were denied recognition as members of the staff of the Western Infirmary, so they could not operate on his behalf. In these circumstances the assistants naturally tended to move on to other posts in which they could acquire direct experience.

During the First World War Macewen acted as Consultant Surgeon to the Navy, caring for naval casualties, and establishing Erskine House as an institute for the manufacture and fitting of artificial limbs. After the war he continued his work as Professor, and in 1922 he was elected President of the British Medical Association. This led in 1923 to a voyage to America and on to Australia, where he fulfilled many engagements. He was tired on his return and he soon succumbed to influenza, from which he died in March 1924.

Macewen's life was one of extraordinary achievement. His reputation was such that it tended to set him apart from his more conventional contemporaries, but his students and house surgeons knew that he had a more human side. Duguid valued a memory from Christmas 1909 when he walked out one evening with Macewen from the Western Infirmary: he was the recipient of wise advice and warm encouragement for his future, whilst they stood on the Dumbarton Road.[50] Then the tramcar arrived, and the tall, impressive figure of Sir William jumped aboard and was borne away to Charing Cross, and his home around the corner in Woodside Crescent.

Lister meanwhile had been working in London and, after his difficult early years, was widely recognised as the pioneer of a revolution in surgery. In 1883 he was knighted by Queen Victoria. He was often called on to address national and international meetings. In 1892 he fulfilled a particularly meaningful engagement when he attended the celebrations of Pasteur's 70th birthday in Paris. There was a great assembly in the Sorbonne, with the main amphitheatre holding some 2,500 people. Lister attended as the representative of the Royal Societies of London and of Edinburgh. Pasteur had never recovered from an earlier stroke, and he had to be helped to his seat by the President of the Republic, who opened the proceedings with a short speech. After other speakers, Lister was called upon and delivered a gracious tribute, in French, in which he gave full weight to the great debt that he personally owed to Pasteur. 'Thanks to you,' he said, 'surgery has undergone a complete revolution, which has deprived it of its terrors, and enlarged almost without limitations its power for good.' Pasteur rose and Lister stepped up to embrace him. The official record likened this to a 'living picture of the brotherhood of science in the relief of humanity'[51] (fig. 7.9).

In 1892, when he was 65, Lister was due to retire from the Chair of Surgery at King's. The staff invited him to stay on for another year, which he was glad to do. His career as clinician and surgeon has been well summed up by Maylard: 'In one sense he may be regarded as a bold surgeon, but his boldness and originality were tempered by good judgement, exercised with discretion and foresight. In the hospital wards it was not only the

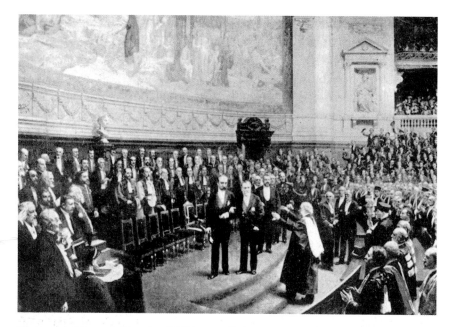

Fig. 7.9. The painting by M. Rixens of the scene in the Sorbonne, Paris, on Pasteur's 70th birthday, 27 December 1892. Following the delivery of his address, Lister walked up the steps to embrace Pasteur. (Godlee, R. J., *Lord Lister*, London, 1917)

healing art that was taught. They – the wards – were a school of gentleness and human sympathy'[52] (fig. 7.10).

In April 1893 Joseph and Agnes set off on a holiday to the Italian Riviera. They enjoyed a week of botanising, but then Agnes caught a chill which speedily developed into pneumonia, which was then a serious condition. Within days Agnes had declined and died, in a hotel room in Rapallo. On that same day, 12 April, Lister sat, enshrouded in grief, and he turned to his friend Cameron, who was himself already a widower: 'I write to you in openness, as we know one another pretty well ... how different life will be to me in the future.' Even so, Lister still remembered to add a postscript: 'I am glad your thumb is well'. (A reference to a septic parrot bite which had disabled Cameron for several months.[53])

There are over a hundred subsequent letters addressed to Cameron and all, right up to the time of Lister's death, are written on notepaper which has a black mourning edging round each

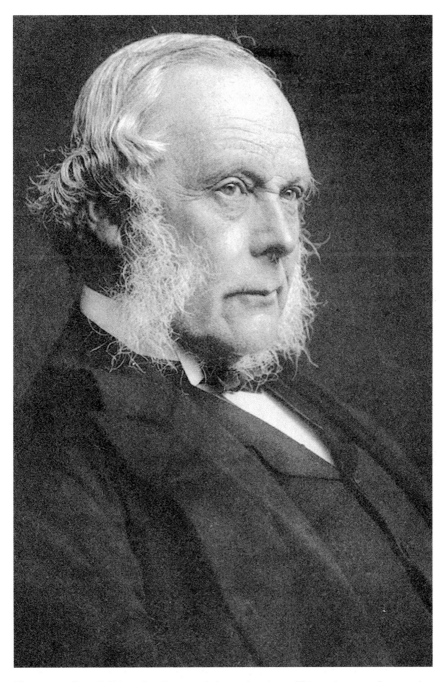

Fig. 7.10. Joseph Lister in 1892, aged 65, at the time of his retirement from active surgery. (Godlee, *Lord Lister*, frontispiece)

sheet. Cameron's son Charles later commented: 'Lister made his wife not only the companion of his leisure but a fellow-worker and critic at his side – it was to Agnes that he clung most and when she died, though he became thereafter increasingly close to my father, all other supports seemed to fail him, leaving him sad, solitary and insecure.'[54] Later, in 1893, the Royal Society appointed Lister to be its Foreign Secretary – an appropriate position for one who had travelled extensively and made many friends abroad. In May 1894 he travelled to Glasgow and stayed with Cameron 'in this hospitable house'. He was due to address the students of the University Medico-Chirurgical Society, where he was received with acclamation. At the close, the students 'must needs unyoke the horse of my cab and draw and push me by a circuitous route to this house', where 'Auld Lang Syne' was sung amid deafening cheers.[55]

In 1895 Lister, who had been elected a Fellow back in 1860, became President of the Royal Society of London. This was only the second time that a doctor of medicine had been so honoured, and Lister welcomed all the occasions when he could meet scientists with so wide a spread of interests.

In the same year he became President of the British Association for the Advancement of Science. At its meeting in Liverpool he spoke on 'The Interdependence of Science and The Healing Art', and for the first time he sought to explain to a lay audience the nature of his own work.[56] Lister told how, after studying Pasteur's observations, he was led to make his own experiment, which had led to real advances in the Healing Art. He then paid tribute to Elie Metchnikoff, of the Pasteur Institute in Paris. In the course of studying starfish in the 1880s he had observed amoeba-like cells which engulfed foreign bodies. This led him to demonstrate that the white corpuscles of mammalian blood likewise included phagocytes, which are a first-line defence against bacterial invasion, and assist in the primary healing of wounds. He then referred to the recent discovery, in 1895, of X-rays. In the course of his experiments, Wilhelm Roentgen, Professor of Physics in Würzburg, Germany, exposed his wife's hand, which lay on a photographic plate, to the radiation from a cathode-ray tube. When developed, the plate showed the structure of the bones of her hand. Lister was not slow to recognise the potential of this discovery. In Aberdeen Dr McKenzie Davidson, Ophthalmologist to the Infirmary, and an experienced photographer, was quick to grasp the importance of Roentgen's discovery, and in his house in Union Street he constructed a cathode-ray tube and began experiments with it. On 14 February 1896 he was able, using a 40-minute exposure, to obtain a radiograph of the foot of a 9-year-old girl containing a broken-off needle. Davidson accurately localised the buried needle and, with Professor Ogston as chloroformist, located and removed it within five minutes.[57] Later that year the Infirmary installed 'Apparatus for Roentgen Skiagraphy', with which Davidson steadily extended his experience.[58] He was visted by radiologists from all over the world, and in 1910 he was chairman of the new Section of Radiology at the meeting of the British Medical Association.

Shortly after Roentgen's discovery came the announcement of another remarkable advance in physics and medicine. In 1895 Marie Sklodowska had married Pierre Curie in Paris, and graduated in physical sciences. In 1897, she began work for a PhD thesis on the properties of uranium. This involved refining sackloads of pitchblende – a time when 'in an old school in the backyard of a Paris school, a woman with a small child, working a man's role and a workman's hours', managed, with Pierre, to isolate the element radium. They described the phenomenon of radioactivity for the first time – the emission of energy arising in the spontaneous activity of sub-atomic particles of an element. For this work the Curies received, with their fellow-worker Becquerel, the 1903 Nobel Prize for Physics.[59]

In 1902 Lister – now Lord Lister – was among the first twelve individuals to be admitted to the Order of Merit, which was established by Edward VII as a personal recognition of achievement. In 1907 Lister's 80th birthday was celebrated. This coincided with the formation of a small group, including Cameron, who set about collecting the papers which had been written by Lister over sixty years. These appeared, in two handsome volumes, as *The Collected Papers of Joseph, Baron Lister*, in 1909.

On his visits south Cameron would call on his old friend and sadly note Lister's slow decline, with sight and hearing slowly deteriorating, until he died in 1912, at the age of 85. The memorial service at Westminster Abbey was thronged up to and beyond the doors, but Lister had insisted that he should be buried beside Agnes in West Hampstead cemetery. At this service the choir sang Handel's anthem which, through a strange blending of texts from the Old and New Testaments, was peculiarly applicable to the occasion:

> When the ear heard him, then it blessed him, and when the eye saw him it gave witness of him; he delivered the poor that cried, the fatherless and him that had none to help him. Kindness, meekness, and comfort were in his tongue. If there was any virtue and if there was any praise, he thought on those things. His body is buried in peace, but his name liveth for evermore.[60]

Hector Cameron was not an innovator, as were his three colleagues – Lister, Ogston and Macewen – although like them he became a Professor of Surgery, was knighted and had a long life. He is especially honoured as a particularly close collaborator and friend of Lister for over forty years. Completely different in character, his warm, outgoing nature and unquestioning support were very important to Lister during the first crucial years of the antisepsis experiment in Glasgow. The friendship thus developed then ripened with the passing years, as Cameron reached maturity and established his own position in Glasgow.

In 1881 he was invited to join the staff of the Western Infirmary, and in 1883 he and Macewen became the first surgeons to the Children's Hospital, which had just commenced work in a large converted town house. Surgical facilities there were few, but their colleague James Nicoll developed a remarkable department at the Dispensary. He was the real pioneer of one-day surgery. Over three years Nicoll performed 406 corrections of hare-lips and cleft palates on infants brought up in the morning, operated on and then taken home in their mothers' arms in the evening. They were then visited for some days by nurses from the Dispensary.[61]

In 1900 Cameron became Professor of Clinical Surgery at the Western Infirmary, retiring from clinical practice in 1911 (fig. 7.11).

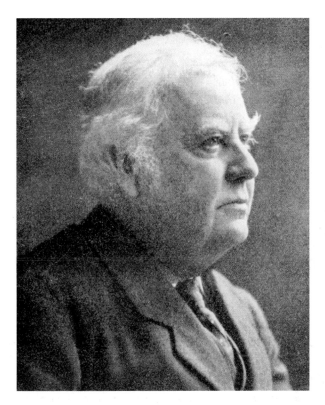

Fig. 7.11. Hector Cameron in 1908, aged 65, at the time of his retirement from the Western Infirmary. (Obituary, *British Medical Journal* 1928, 2: 1015)

Over many years he was elected and re-elected as Dean of Faculties in the University, and for fifteen years he represented Glasgow on the General Medical Council in London. Throughout World War I Sir Hector was the Red Cross Commissioner for the West of Scotland: he had to put to best use nearly 3,000 beds – a task which gave full scope to his tact and judgment. Among all these beds there was one ward of special interest, for part of the Surgical Block of the old Glasgow Royal Infirmary was still standing. This included the historic Ward 24, where Lister had conducted his first trial of antiseptic treatment in 1865–67 (fig. 3.3). Between 1905 and 1914 the old buildings of the Infirmary were steadily demolished while the new Infirmary building was proceeding on the same site. The western half of the old Surgical Hospital was, however, left standing within the forecourt of the new building (fig. 7.12). During the 1914–18 war this old Surgical Hospital block was brought back into use, to accommodate wounded servicemen.

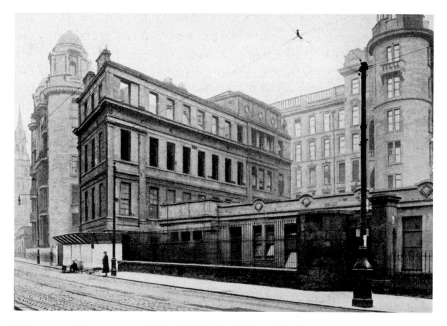

Fig. 7.12. The remnant of the old Surgical Hospital of 1861, still standing in the forecourt of the new Glasgow Royal Infirmary, as it appeared at the time of its demolition in 1924. The white hoarding conceals Ward 24, Lister's male accident ward. (Maylard, 'Lister', in *Lister and the Lister Ward*, Glasgow, 1927.)

In 1919 great controversy arose over the fate of this block, with Sir Hector and many others campaigning for the preservation of historic Ward 24. Eventually they were defeated and the block was demolished in 1924.[62]

In 1921 the General Medical Council judged Sir Hector – then 78 years of age – to be the best man to act as Supervisor of Medical School Examinations throughout Great Britain and Northern Ireland. Cameron travelled throughout the land, and Professor Grey Turner recalled his experience when he was an external examiner in Sheffield. Sir Hector 'spent practically the whole day with the examiners, was often at my elbow, and I felt I was going through a severe ordeal'. Later, Cameron the raconteur was the life and soul of the examiners' dinner.[63]

As the year 1927 approached, the University arranged a celebration of the centenary of the birth of Lister. Cameron's memories were stirred and the result was the publication of his

Reminiscences of Lister.[64] This is a unique account of the time when Cameron worked with Lister between 1865 and 1867. In 45 pages it gives many details of their experiences, with a series of anecdotes. One tells of the occasion when Lister and Cameron had driven to the Infirmary in Lister's brougham. The coachman was asked to wait on the driveway, while Lister and Cameron were in Ward 24, on the ground floor of the Surgical Hospital. The waiting horses grew restless, and suddenly there was a great cry from outside the ward. Then came the sound of carriage and horses crashing and overturning, down into the deep area in front of the basement. Lister dashed out, and down the slope. The night was dark and cold, the carriage lay on its side, while the whinnying, terrified horses thrashed their legs, striking sparks off the wall of the basement. The horses lay between Lister and his coachman, who was pinned under the carriage. For a moment the kicking ceased, and Lister leapt across the horses' legs and, helping to lift the carriage, released the coachman and carried him into the ward. The only fracture was a broken arm, but the man was complaining bitterly of abdominal pain, and examination showed the signs of peritonitis. Lister suspected that a blow on the abdomen had ruptured part of the intestines but in the 1860s 'it was considered almost criminal to open the abdomen intentionally'.[65] The coachman died from spreading peritonitis, and the autopsy confirmed that there was a small tear in the wall of the small intestine, with consequent leakage of bowel content into the abdomen. It would be another forty years before surgeons regularly opened the abdomen for such accidental injuries, often finding that it was a simple matter to suture the hole in the bowel wall, wash out the abdomen, and anticipate a quick recovery.

In 1929, after a short illness, Cameron died at the age of 86. His name is inseparably associated with Lister, for good reasons, but beyond this productive partnership Cameron led an unusually full and long professional life, and his friends remembered other interests: 'he was widely read, and remembered what he had read. He was as observant on the hillside, on the links and beside the river as he was amongst his patients. He loved tracking the birds and identifying the various callers. He leaves a happy memory, gracious and inspiring.'[66]

Lister was not a Scot, but he achieved the crucial breakthrough in the conquest of surgical sepsis during the twenty years that he worked in Scotland. He was supported by a remarkable team. First, there was the faithful Cameron, then Ogston working in his garden laboratory provided the essential bacteriological evidence. Then came the polymath Macewen, bombarding his colleagues with fresh evidence of the potential of aseptic surgery. Alongside was Thomas Keith, steadily building up evidence that meticulous cleanliness matters, and James Simpson with his discovery of chloroform. The Scottish Enlightenment of the eighteenth century is well recognised. Scotland can also fairly claim to have made the major contribution to the enlightenment which transformed surgical practice in the nineteenth century.

Chronology

1789	French Revolution
1792	Coal gas used for street lighting
1795	Alexander Gordon, Aberdeen – monograph on puerperal fever
1797	Edward Jenner: monograph on vaccination against smallpox
1799	James Syme born (d. 1870)
	Humphry Davy: anaesthetic properties of nitrous oxide
1805	Battle of Trafalgar
1809	Ephraim McDowell: first recorded ovariotomy, Kentucky, USA
1811	J. Y. Simpson born (d. 1870)
1815	Battle of Waterloo
	Jane Austen, *Pride and Prejudice*
1821	James Syme graduated
1827	Joseph Lister born (d. 1912)
	Thomas Keith, Edinburgh, born (d. 1895)
1830	Liverpool–Manchester railway opened
1831–32	First major cholera epidemic in UK
1832	Great Reform Bill
	Surgical Hospital, Edinburgh Royal Infirmary, opened
1833	James Syme appointed Professor of Surgery, Edinburgh
	Factory Acts: limits on child labour
1837	Accession of Queen Victoria
1838	William Keith appointed Surgeon to Aberdeen Royal Infirmary.

1840		Simpson building, Aberdeen Royal Infirmary, opened
		Penny Post
1843		Hector Cameron born (d. 1929)
1844		Alexander Ogston born (d. 1929)
1845		Lawson Tait born (d. 1899)
1846, October		William Morton administered ether, Massachusetts General Hospital
	December	Liston/Squire: ether anaesthesia at University College Hospital, London
1847, November		J. Y. Simpson: chloroform anaesthesia, Edinburgh
1848		William Macewen born (d. 1924)
1850		Charles Dickens, *David Copperfield*
1851		Joseph Lister qualified, University College Hospital, London
		Great Exhibition, Hyde Park, London
1853, September		Joseph Lister arrived in Edinburgh
1854		Joseph Lister, House Surgeon to Professor Syme
1854–56		Crimean War
1856		Agnes Syme and Joseph Lister married
1857		Spencer Wells: first report on ovariotomy, London
1858		Indian Mutiny
1859		Loch Katrine, water aqueduct to Glasgow opened
		Charles Darwin, *On the Origin of Species*
1860		J. Lister appointed Professor of Surgery, University of Glasgow
		J. Lister elected Fellow, Royal Society of London
1860–65		American Civil War
1861, May		Surgical Hospital, Glasgow Royal Infirmary, opened
	August	J. Lister, Surgeon to Glasgow Royal Infirmary
	December	Albert, Prince Consort, died
1862		Thomas Keith: first ovariotomy, Edinburgh
1865		J. Lister: commenced antiseptic treatment of compound fractures
		Alexander Ogston graduated, Aberdeen
		Assassination of Abraham Lincoln
1867		J. Lister: first paper on the Antiseptic Principle
		Hector Cameron: House Surgeon, then Assistant, to Lister

1869	Professor Syme suffered stroke
	J. Lister: Professor of Clinical Surgery, University of Edinburgh
	Leo Tolstoy, *War and Peace*
	Suez Canal opened
1870	Franco-Prussian War
1872	Scottish Education Act
	George Eliot, *Middlemarch*
1873	Hector Cameron, Surgeon to Glasgow Royal Infirmary
1874	Alexander Ogston, Full Surgeon, Aberdeen Royal Infirmary
1876	A. Ogston: first osteotomy for knock-knee
	William Macewen, Full Surgeon, Glasgow Royal Infirmary
	Queen Victoria created Empress of India
	Graham Bell and the telephone
1877	J. Lister appointed Professor of Surgery, King's College, London
1879	Thomas Keith completed 300 ovariotomies, Edinburgh
1879–81	A. Ogston: bacteriological experiments: *Staphylococcus aureus*
1881	W. Macewen: first neurosurgical paper
	Theodor Billroth: first gastrectomy for cancer, Vienna
1882	A. Ogston: Regius Professor of Surgery, University of Aberdeen
1883	Lawson Tait: first successful operation for ruptured ectopic pregnancy
	Daimler-Benz: internal combustion engine
1884	William Macewen reported 700 patients undergoing osteotomy
	Neuber, Kiel: operating theatre for 'aseptic' surgery
1886	R. Fitz: pathology and diagnosis of acute appendicitis
1888	William Macewen: address on 'Surgery of the Brain and Spinal Cord'
1889	Charles McBurney: clinical picture and treatment of acute appendicitis

1892	Louis Pasteur: 70th birthday, meeting with Lister in Sorbonne, Paris
	William Macewen: Regius Professor of Surgery, University of Glasgow
	Heusner: first successful suture of perforated gastric ulcer
1893	Death of Agnes Lister
	Retirement of Joseph Lister
1895	Lister elected President, Royal Society of London
	Roentgen discovered X-rays
	Marconi and wireless telegraphy
1898	The Curies discover radium
	First diesel engine
1899–1902	Boer War
1900	Hector Cameron: Professor of Surgery, University of Glasgow
1901	Death of Queen Victoria
1902	Lister admitted to Order of Merit
	Edward VII: acute appendicitis
1903	Wright Brothers: first powered flight
1909	The *Collected Papers of Joseph Baron Lister* published in two volumes
1910	Death of Edward VII
	Accession of George V
1911	Lloyd George's National Insurance Act
1912	Death of Lord Lister
1914	Outbreak of First World War
1916	A. Ogston: medical officer on the Italian Front
1918, November	Armistice
1924	Death of Macewen
	First Labour Government
1927	Hector Cameron published *Reminiscences of Lister*
1929	Deaths of Ogston and Cameron

Glossary

Abscess. A localised collection of pus, due to bacterial infection. This can occur anywhere in the body. It may be acute and painful, needing drainage, or a chronic collection, as in a tuberculous psoas abscess.

Amyloid disease. Infiltration of tissues, especially liver, spleen and kidneys, with a waxy material, amyloid. Now rare, this was seen as a chronic debilitating condition, resulting from long-continued sepsis, such as lung abscess or chronic osteomyelitis.

Aneurysm. A saccular enlargement of an artery, due to weakening of its wall.

Ankylosis. Fixity of a joint, due to accidental injury, or disease.

Aorta/Artery. The aorta arises from the left ventricle of the heart and carries oxygenated blood to all parts of the body. It first forms the aortic arch, from which arise the *carotid* arteries, supplying the head and neck, and the *axillary* arteries supplying the arms. The thoracic aorta then descends through the left chest, supplying the rib cage, and passes through the diaphragm, becoming the *abdominal aorta*. This supplies the abdominal organs and the lower part of the body. It bifurcates in the pelvis to form the two *iliac* arteries, one to each leg. Beneath the groin, as it enters the leg, the *external iliac* becomes the *femoral* artery which runs down close to the femur. Above and behind the knee joint, the femoral becomes the *popliteal* artery, which in turn, beyond the knee, divides into the *tibial* arteries.

In the arm, the *axillary* artery (in the armpit) then becomes the *brachial* as far as the elbow, where it divides into the *radial* and *ulnar* arteries, which supply the forearm and hand.

Appendix. Vestigial organ, 5–8 cm long, arising from the lower pole of caecum.

Articular surfaces. The smooth, cartilaginous surfaces over the bones of a joint, which allow easy movement on each other.

Ascitic fluid. Fluid accumulated within the abdominal cavity in various diseases.

Autoclave. An apparatus for sterilising surgical linen, dressings and instruments by the admission of steam under pressure into a reinforced metal chamber. Exposure of the contents to a temperature of 120–130°C for 15 minutes kills all organisms.

Bacteraemia. The presence of bacteria in the blood – this is due to 'overflow' from an infective condition, but it is not one in which active multiplication of bacteria occurs (cf. *Septicaemia*).

Bile duct. The duct which leads from the liver to the small intestine, delivering bile. If a stone obstructs the duct, jaundice is likely to appear.

Boil. A minor abscess, often due to infection arising in a hair follicle.

Caecum. The first part of the large intestine: the appendix arises from its lower pole.

Carbuncle. An acute and often serious staphylococcal infection, spreading in the skin and subcutaneous tissues on the back of the neck. It commonly shows several openings.

Caries. Decay of a bone. As used in the past, this was another name for tuberculous disease of bone.

Carpal and metacarpal bones. Bones at the wrist. The carpus is a collection of eight small bones, between the lower end of the ulna and the five metacarpal bones. The metacarpals can be felt on the back of the palm, and articulate with the thumb and four fingers.

Cellulitis. An acute, painful infection within tissues. Most commonly seen in the skin and subcutaneous tissues as a red, swollen, tender area; especially severe in *erysipelas*, an acute streptococcal infection of the skin, with a well-defined and advancing red edge.

Colon or large intestine. Joins the small intestine to the rectum.

Compound fracture. A fracture of a bone which communicates with an open wound in the overlying skin and tissues.

Condyle. Expanded, shaped, swellings at the inner and outer ends of femur and tibia, which bear weight and movement at the joint.

Craniotomy. Opening or cutting the skull. In an obstetric context the operation is now very rare. In rickets, with a deformed pelvis, with consequent obstructed labour, it was necessary to incise and crush the skull of the dead baby before its extraction.

Delirium tremens. An acute psychotic state occurring in some chronic alcoholics, particularly when alcohol intake is suddenly withdrawn.

Diaphragm. A domed muscle, separating thorax from abdomen.

Duodenum. Short, c-shaped, first part of small intestine, joining stomach to jejunum.

Dura mater. The tough outermost covering of the brain and spinal cord.

Emphysema. The state in which tissues are distended with air. Surgical emphysema occurs when air lies in tissues beneath the skin, giving a crackling feeling.

Empyema. Pus has accumulated within a space (e.g. the pleural cavity) or an organ, for example in empyema of the gall bladder.

Entozoa. Intestinal parasites of animals.

Epiglottis. Lid-like structure, which protects the entrance to the larynx.

Erysipelas. See *Cellulitis.*

Fallopian tube, or oviduct. The fringed open ends of the oviducts lie adjacent to the ovaries: they receive eggs shed from the ovaries and conduct them to the uterus.

Femur. The thigh bone, extending from the hip joint to the knee joint.

Fibula. Slender bone in the leg, lying on outer side of the tibia.

Fistula. An abnormal opening between one hollow organ and another, or between a hollow organ, (e.g. intestine or gall bladder) and the skin, with consequent external faecal or biliary discharge. May be the result of injury, disease or a congenital malformation.

Gall bladder. Part of the biliary tract, where bile is stored. This is the usual site for the formation of gallstones.

Graves' disease, or thyrotoxicosis. Named after Robert Graves (1796–1853), Irish physician. A state of overactivity of the thyroid gland, with an excess of circulating thyroid hormone. This produces hyperactivity, loss of weight, overaction of the heart and exophthalmos (protrusion of the eyeball).

Greater trochanter. The part of the femur just below the hip joint. It can be felt below the hard edge of the bony pelvis.

Hospital gangrene. A form of wound infection, which was a serious problem in pre-antiseptic days. It attacked any open wound, which became blackened and covered in grey sloughs. Very difficult to eradicate, even leading to amputation of a limb.

Humerus. Bone of the upper arm, lying between the shoulder joint and the elbow.

Hydrocele. Swelling of the scrotum due to fluid surrounding the testis.

Intestines. Small intestine is a smooth tube, 2 cm diameter, 6–7 metres long, lying in the centre of the abdomen, and joining the stomach and duodenum to the colon.

Large intestine. See *Colon.*

Larynx. The voice box, which can be felt high in the neck, in mid-line. Below it joins onto the trachea, or windpipe, which can be felt in the mid-line until it enters the chest. The operation of tracheotomy opens the trachea just below the larynx

Ligature. A length of silk, linen thread or catgut, which should be sterile, tied around a vessel to arrest bleeding.

Lithotrity. Crushing of a stone in the bladder by an instrument passed up the urethra.

Mastectomy. Operative removal of the breast.

Mesmerism. A form of hypnotism introduced by F. A. Mesmer (1735–1810), Austrian physician. The subject usually lost consciousness, and was sometimes insensitive to pain. A colleague of Liston's had been using mesmerism in surgical patients, but it had not provided reliable relief from the pain of surgery.

Micrococci. Micro-organisms which, on staining, appear as bunches (staphylococci) or in chains (streptococci).

Osteomyelitis. An acute staphylococcal infection of bone, which affects both the shaft and the marrow. Until the arrival of penicillin, this was a not-uncommon and dangerous disease, causing high fever and acute pain, progressing to septicaemia. An emergency operation was required to drill the bone and release pus under tension. Without antibiotics, this disease often became chronic, with separation of pieces of bone.

Osteotome. A chisel specially designed to cut through bone, in the operation of osteotomy. This allowed correction of bony deformities.

Ovariotomy. The removal of a large cyst of the ovary, by open abdominal operation.

Peptic ulcer. A breach of the lining mucous membrane of the stomach or duodenum, usually due to over-secretion of acid and pepsin.

Perineum. In males, the area immediately behind the scrotum and in front of the anus.

Perineal lithotomy. Involved an incision across this area, which led up by dissection to the back of the bladder, which was opened and a stone removed.

Peritoneal cavity. Cavity of the abdomen, lined by the glistening, lubricating, peritoneal membrane. This allows free movement to organs such as stomach and intestines.

Peritonitis. A dangerous infection of the peritoneal cavity, usually due to perforation of a hollow organ, e.g. perforation of a peptic ulcer, or perforated acute appendicitis. Also occurs if an abdominal wound punctures a hollow organ.

Phthisis. The word derives from the Greek, meaning 'to waste away'. In practice this word came to be synonymous with pulmonary tuberculosis.

Popliteal aneurysm. Widening of the artery behind the knee joint.

Pott's disease. Tuberculosis of the spine, associated with destruction of a vertebral body, with consequent angulation. Named after Percivall Pott, eighteenth-century surgeon.

Prostate. Gland surrounding male urethra immediately below bladder.

Psoas abscess. In tuberculosis of the spine the affected vertebra(e) are surrounded by an abscess which spreads, behind the abdominal cavity, to present in the groin.

Pubis. Central part of bony pelvic ring, to be felt above root of penis.

Pyaemia. A bacterial infection in which the sepsis involves a vein, causing clotting. This breaks down and is spread via the venous circulation to cause multiple abscesses.

Putrefaction. Decomposition of animal or vegetable matter by micro-organisms, accompanied by the production of gases with an offensive smell.

Radius and ulna. The bones of the forearm.

Scrofula. An outdated name for tuberculosis of lymph glands, especially in the neck.

Septicaemia. Pathogenic micro-organisms are actively multiplying in the bloodstream, producing a serious illness, with high fever and shivering fits.

Sequestrum. Dead piece of bone, sequel to infection, lying within long bone, and acting as a foreign body.

Struma. An archaic term meaning a swelling in the neck. Usually refers to a swelling of the thyroid (goitre), but also synonymous with scrofula.

Tibia. The shin-bone.

Trachea. See *Larynx*.

Trench foot. This was often seen in the First World War, among troops who were standing for long periods in cold, waterlogged trenches. A form of frostbite, with gangrene, due partly to temperature and partly to poor circulation caused by lack of exercise.

Tuberculosis. Any infection by the tubercle bacillus: there are two strains of the organism. The bovine form, caused by *Mycobacterium tuberculosis bovis*, was spread by drinking raw milk from a cow with an affected udder. Before pasteurization, this was a common cause of disease, particularly in children, in bones and joints, and in lymph glands, especially in the neck.

The human form is mostly spread from person to person by inhalation, a main cause of pulmonary tuberculosis.

Typhlitis. An outdated term, meaning inflammation of the caecum, which fell into disuse when it was realized that the true source of the inflammation was the appendix.

Ureter. Tube which transfers urine from kidney to bladder.

Urethra. The channel along which urine passes from the bladder to the exterior.

Urethral staff. A smooth, curved rod with a rounded tip, which was passed along the urethra into the bladder: it had a groove on the lower aspect of the curve. The term 'urethral sound' dates from the days before X-rays. Then, a stone in the bladder was diagnosed on its symptoms, and on the fact that when a urethral staff or sound was passed into the bladder, the impact of the tip of the instrument touching a stone could be felt and heard. With experience, the size of the stone could be estimated.

Notes

Chapter 1: Surgery before Anaesthesia and Antisepsis, 1837–1845

1. Turner, A. L., *The Story of a Great Hospital: the Royal Infirmary of Edinburgh, 1729–1929* (Edinburgh, 1937): 180–200.
2. Shepherd, J. A., *Simpson and Syme of Edinburgh* (Edinburgh, 1969): 23–4.
3. Wangensteen, O. H. and Wangensteen, S. D., *The Rise of Surgery* (Folkestone, 1978): 36.
4. Syme, J., *Edinburgh Medical Surgical Journal* 1824, 21: 19–27.
5. *Ibid.*
6. *Ibid.*
7. White, H., 'Surgery in the eighteenth and nineteenth centuries', in Medvei, V. C. and Thornton, J. L., eds, *The Royal Hospital of St Bartholomew, 1123–1973* (London, 1974): 207.
8. Peddie, A., *Edinburgh Medical Journal* 1890, 35: 1048–62.
9. Brogden, W. A., *Aberdeen: An Architectural Guide* (Edinburgh, 1986): 35–55.
10. *Ibid.*
11. Mackenzie, H., *The City of Aberdeen* (Edinburgh, Third Statistical Survey, 1953).
12. Levack, I. D. and Dudley, H. A. F., *Aberdeen Royal Infirmary* (London, 1992): 90.
13. Woodham-Smith, C., *Florence Nightingale* (London, 1950): 57–8.
14. Ogston, A., 'How antiseptic surgery came to Aberdeen', in Ogston, W. H., ed., *Alexander Ogston, KCVO* (Aberdeen, 1943): 93.
15. Annual Reports, Aberdeen Royal Infirmary, 1840–44.
16. Ogston, A. 'How antiseptic surgery came to Aberdeen': 93.
17. Crosse, V. M., *A Surgeon in the Early Nineteenth Century: the life and times of John Green Crosse, 1790–1850* (Edinburgh, 1968).
18. *Ibid.*
19. Keith, W., *Edinburgh Medical Journal* 1844, 61: 396–417.
20. *Ibid.*
21. *Ibid.*
22. *Ibid.*
23. *Ibid.*
24. *Ibid.*: 123–9.

25. *Ibid.*
26. Cope, V. Z., *William Cheselden, 1688–1752* (Edinburgh, 1953): 29.
27. Adam, L., personal communication.
28. Thompson, H., 'William Keith', *Lancet* 1871, 1: 289.
29. Godlee, R. J., *Lord Lister* (London, 1917): 35.

Chapter 2: The Arrival of General Anaesthesia, 1846–1860

1. Fulton, J. F., *Anesthesiology* 1947, 8: 464–70.
2. *Ibid.*
3. Rushman, G. B. *et al.*, *A Short History of Anaesthesia* (Oxford, 1996): 9–19.
4. *Ibid.*
5. Boland, F. K., *Surgery* 1943, 13: 270–81.
6. *Ibid.*
7. *Ibid.*
8. Editorial, 'The discovery of nitrous oxide and ether', *British Medical Journal* (hereafter *BMJ*) 1896, 2: 1137–40.
9. Vandam, L. D. and Abbott, J. A., *New England Journal of Medicine* 1984, 311: 991–4.
10. Eavey, R. D., *New England Journal of Medicine* 1983, 309: 990–1.
11. Bigelow, H. J., 'Surgical operations performed during insensibility', *Lancet* 1847, 1: 6–8.
12. *Ibid.*
13. Morton, W. T. G., *Lancet* 1847, 2: 80–1.
14. *Ibid.*
15. Bigelow, H. J., 'Surgical operations performed during insensibility', *Lancet* 1847, 1: 6–8.
16. Bigelow, J., *Lancet* 1847, 1: 5–6.
17. Ellis, R. H., *Anaesthesia* 1977, 32: 197–208.
18. *Ibid.*
19. Ellis, R. H., *Anaesthesia* 1976, 31: 766–77.
20. Bigelow, J., *Lancet* 1847, 1: 5–6.
21. Bigelow, H. J., 'Surgical operations performed during insensibility', *Lancet* 1847, 1: 6–8.
22. Squire, W., 'On the introduction of ether inhalation as an anaesthetic in London', *Lancet* 1888, 2: 1220–1.
23. Zuck, D., *British Journal of Anaesthesia* 1978, 50: 393–405.
24. *Ibid.*
25. Squire, 'On the introduction of ether inhalation': 1220–1.
26. Dawkins, C. J. M., *Anaesthesia* 1947, 2: 51–61.
27. *Ibid.*
28. Squire, 'On the introduction of ether inhalation': 1220–1.
29. *Ibid.*
30. *Ibid.*
31. Liston, R., quoted by Boott, F., *Lancet* 1847, 1: 8.
32. Shepard, J. A., *Simpson and Syme of Edinburgh* (Edinburgh, 1969): 83–5.

33. Hovell, B.C. and Wilson J., *Journal of the Royal College of Surgeons of Edinburgh* 1969, 14: 107–16.

34. Baillie, T.W., *From Boston to Dumfries* (Dumfries, 1966): 1–32.

35. Scott, W., *Lancet* 1872, 2: 585.

36. *Ibid.*

37. Editorial, *Aberdeen Journal*, 10 February 1847.

38. Rushman *et al.*, *A Short History of Anaesthesia*: 9–19.

39. Furnell, M.C., *Lancet* 1877, 1: 934–6.

40. Simpson, D., *Scottish Medical Journal* 1990, 35: 451–5.

41. Duncan, I., *Memoir of Dr James M. Duncan* (Aberdeen Medico-Chirurgical Society, 1891).

42. Simpson, D., *Scottish Medical Journal* 1990, 35: 451–5.

43. Simpson, J.Y., *Lancet* 1847, 2: 549–50.

44. Lister, J., 'On anaesthesia', in *Collected Papers* (Oxford, 1909), I: 135–60.

45. Keith, W., *Monthly Journal of Medical Science* (1848–49).

46. Hill, A.B., *Proceedings of the Royal Society of Medicine* 1955, 48: 1008–12.

47. Longford, E., *Victoria RI* (London, 1966): 291–2.

48. MacWilliam, J.A., *BMJ* 1890, 2: 948–50.

49. Editorial, 'Ether vs. chloroform', *BMJ* 1872, 2: 499–501.

50. Godlee, R.J., *Lord Lister* (London, 1917): 1–15.

51. Lister, J., 'Address to British Association, 1896', in *Collected Papers* (Oxford, 1909), II: 489–514.

52. Keiller, A., *Edinburgh Medical Journal* 1884, 29: 984.

53. Godlee, *Lord Lister*, 30–42.

54. *Ibid.*

55. Turner, A.L., *Story of a Great Hospital: Royal Infirmary of Edinburgh, 1729–1929* (Edinburgh, 1937): 206–8, 168.

56. Syme, J., *Lancet* 1 (1855): 55–7.

57. Godlee, *Lord Lister*: 30–42.

58. *Ibid.*: 57–66.

59. Learmonth, J., *Scottish Medical Journal* 2003, 48: 125–6.

60. Fisher, R., *Joseph Lister, 1827–1912* (London, 1977): 187.

61. Godlee, *Lord Lister*: 91.

62. Fisher, *Joseph Lister*: 103.

Chapter 3: The Path Towards Antisepsis, 1795–1865

1. Loudon, I., *The Tragedy of Childbed Fever* (Oxford, 2000): 24–35.

2. Porter, I.A., *Alexander Gordon of Aberdeen, 1752–1799* (Edinburgh, 1958).

3. Colebrook, L., 'The story of puerperal fever, 1800–1950', *BMJ* 1956, 1: 247–52.

4. Porter, *Alexander Gordon of Aberdeen*.

5. *Ibid.*

6. *Ibid.*

7. Holmes, O.W., 'The contagiousness of puerperal fever', *New England Quarterly Journal of Medicine and Surgery* 1843, 1: 503–30.

8. *Ibid.*
9. Colebrook, 'The story of puerperal fever': 247–52.
10. *Ibid.*
11. Simpson, J.Y., *Monthly Journal of Medical Science* 1850, 2: 414–29.
12. *Ibid.*
13. *Ibid.*
14. Simpson, J.Y., *Monthly Journal of Medical Science* 1851, 4: 72–80.
15. Loudon, I., *The Tragedy of Childbed Fever*: 116, 139, 144.
16. *Ibid.*
17. Doleris, J.A., *La Fièvre Puerperal* (Paris, 1880).
18. Colebrook, 'The story of puerperal fever': 247–52.
19. Macfarlane, G., *Alexander Fleming* (Oxford, 1985): 127–76.
20. Colebrook, 'The story of puerperal fever': 247–52.
21. Macfarlane, *Alexander Fleming*: 127–76.
22. *Ibid.*
23. Peddie, A., *Edinburgh Medical Journal* 1890, 35: 1048–62.
24. Keith, T., 'Fifty-one cases of ovariotomy', *Lancet* 1867, 2: 290–1.
25. Lizars, J., *Edinburgh Medical and Surgical Journal* 1824, 22: 247–56.
26. *Ibid.*
27. Shepherd, J.A., *Spencer Wells* (Edinburgh, 1965): 41–52, 97.
28. Leading article, 'Ovariotomy', *BMJ* 1880, 1: 931–2.
29. Shepherd, *Spencer Wells*: 41–52, 97.
30. Wells, T.S., *Lancet* 1872, 2: 814–15.
31. Shepherd, *Spencer Wells*: 41–52, 97.
32. 'Ovariotomy', *BMJ*: 931–2.
33. Obituary, Thomas Keith, *Lancet* 1895, 2: 1014–15.
34. *Ibid.*
35. Keith, T., 'Fifty-one cases of ovariotomy': 290–1.
36. *Ibid.*
37. Obituary, Thomas Keith: 1014–15.
38. Skene, A.J.C., 'Thomas Keith', *Brooklyn Medical Journal* 1896, 10: 73–80.
39. Obituary, Thomas Keith: 1014–15.
40. Keith, T., 'Fifty-one cases of ovariotomy': 290–1.
41. Skene, A.J.C., 'Thomas Keith', *Brooklyn Medical Journal* 1896, 10: 73–80.
42. Keith, 'Fifty-one cases of ovariotomy': 290–1.
43. Keith, T., *Lancet* 1870, 2: 249–51.
44. Shepherd, *Spencer Wells*: 41–52, 97.
45. Keith, T., *Lancet* 1878, 2: 590–3.
46. Sims, J.M., *American Journal of Obstetrics and Diseases of Women and Children* 1880, 13: 290–303.
47. Leading article, 'A great deed in surgery', *BMJ* 1879, 2: 915–16.
48. Shepherd, J.A., *Lawson Tait: The Rebellious Surgeon* (Lawrence, Kansas, 1980).
49. *Ibid.*

50. Keith, T., *Lancet* 1878, 2: 590–3.
51. Fisher, R., *Joseph Lister, 1827–1912* (London, 1977): 100.
52. Godlee, R.J., *Lord Lister* (London, 1917): 92.
53. Robertson, E., *Glasgow's Doctor: J. B. Russell, 1834–1904* (East Linton, 1998): 198.
54. Jenkinson, J. *et al. The Royal: The History of the Glasgow Royal Infirmary, 1794–1994* (Glasgow, 1994).
55. Godlee, *Lord Lister*: 92.
56. Lister, J., *Lancet* 1870, 1: 4–6.
57. Cameron, H.C., *Reminiscences of Lister and his Work in the Glasgow Royal Infirmary, 1860–1869* (Glasgow, 1927): 11–12.
58. *Collected Papers of Joseph, Baron Lister* (Oxford, 1909), Introduction: XIII.
59. Fisher, *Joseph Lister*: 125.
60. Devine, T.M., *Exploring the Scottish Past* (East Linton, 1995): 129–30.
61. Robertson, *Glasgow's Doctor: J. B. Russell*.
62. Lister, J., *Lancet* 1870, 1: 4–6.
63. Cameron, *Reminiscences of Lister*: 11–12.
64. Lister, J., 'On excision of the wrist for caries', *Lancet* 1865, 1: 308–12, 335–8, 362–4.
65. *Ibid.*
66. *Ibid.*
67. *Ibid.*
68. Fisher, *Joseph Lister*: 112.
69. *Ibid.*: 101–2.
70. *Ibid.*

Chapter 4: The Birth of the Antiseptic Principle, 1867–1870

1. Lister, J., *Lancet* 1867, 2: 353–6.
2. *Collected Papers of Joseph, Baron Lister* (Oxford, 1909), Introduction: XII.
3. Lister, J., *Lancet* 1867, 2: 353–6.
4. Lister, J., *BMJ* 1871, 2: 225–33.
5. *Ibid.*
6. Lister, J., *Lancet* 1867, 1: 326–9, 357–9, 387–8, 507–9.
7. *Ibid.*
8. *Ibid.*
9. *Ibid.*
10. *Ibid.*
11. *Ibid.*
12. Lister, J., *Lancet* 1867, 2: 353–6.
13. Godlee, R.J., *Lord Lister* (London, 1917): 192–4.
14. Lister, J., *Lancet* 1867, 1: 326–9, 357–9, 387–8, 507–9.
15. Lister, J., *Lancet* 1867, 2: 353–6.
16. *Ibid.*
17. *Ibid.*

18. Lister, J., Lettter to William Macewen, 24 November 1877. In Macewen Archive, Royal College of Physicians and Surgeons, Glasgow.
19. Cameron, H. Clare, *Reminiscences of Lord Lister* (Glasgow, 1927): 28–30.
20. *Ibid.*
21. Godlee, *Lord Lister*: 213.
22. Cameron, *Reminiscences of Lord Lister*: 28–30.
23. Lister, J., *Edinburgh Medical Journal* 1875, 21: 193–205.
24. *Collected Papers of Joseph, Baron Lister*, vol. 2: 63.
25. Cameron, H. Charles, *Joseph Lister: the friend of man* (London, 1948): 6, 64, 67.
26. Lister, J., *BMJ* 1868, 2: 53–6.
27. Cameron, *Joseph Lister: the friend of man*: 6, 64, 67.
28. Cameron, *Reminiscences of Lord Lister*: 17–19.
29. Lister, J., *Lancet* 1869, 1: 451–5.
30. Godlee, *Lord Lister*, 231.
31. Fisher, R., *Lord Lister, 1827–1912* (London, 1977): 166.
32. Lister, J., *Lancet* 1869, 1: 451–5.
33. Bickersteth, E. R., *Lancet* 1869, 1: 743–4, 811–12.
34. Lister, Lord, *Lancet* 1908, 1: 148.
35. Cresswell, P. R., *Lancet* 1868, 2: 277.
36. Lister, J., *Lancet* 1870, 2: 287–9.
37. Godlee, *Lord Lister*: 353–4.
38. *Ibid.*
39. Cameron, *Joseph Lister: the friend of man*: 6, 64, 67.
40. Cameron, *Reminiscences of Lord Lister*: 43–4.
41. Godlee, *Lord Lister*: 241–3.
42. *Ibid.*
43. Daiches, D., *Glasgow* (London, 1977): 153–4.
44. Mackie, J. E., *The University of Glasgow, 1451–1951* (Glasgow, 1954): 277, 280.
45. *Ibid.*
46. Lister, J., *Lancet* 1870, 1: 4–6, 40–2.
47. *Ibid.*
48. Lister, J., *Lancet* 1867, 2: 353–6.
49. Lamond, H., *Lancet* 1870, 1: 175.
50. Lister, J., *Lancet* 1870, 1: 4–6, 40–2.
51. Lamond, H., *Lancet* 1870, 1: 175.
52. Godlee, *Lord Lister*: 251.

Chapter 5: Development of the Antiseptic Principle, 1870–1880

1. Lister, J., *BMJ* 1871, 2: 225–33.
2. Turner, A. L., *The Story of a Great Hospital: The Royal Infirmary of Edinburgh, 1729–1929* (Edinburgh, 1937): 239–40.
3. Lister, J., *BMJ* 1871, 2: 225–33.
4. *Ibid.*

5. Leeson, J. R., *Lister as I Knew Him* (London, 1927), 16–24.

6. *Ibid.*: 48–55.

7. *Ibid.*

8. *Ibid.*

9. *Ibid.*: 16–24.

10. *Ibid.*: 48–55.

11. *Ibid.*

12. Godlee, R. J., *Lord Lister* (London, 1917): 259.

13. *Ibid.*

14. Leeson, J. R., *Lister as I Knew Him*: 105–20.

15. Godlee, *Lord Lister*: 600.

16. Lister, J., *BMJ* 1871, 1: 30–2.

17. Leeson, J. R., *Lister as I Knew Him*: 105–20.

18. Lister J., *BMJ* 1890, 2: 377–9.

19. Cameron, H. Charles, *Joseph Lister, the friend of man* (London, 1948): 9.

20. Lister, J., *BMJ* 1908, 2: 1557–8.

21. *Ibid.*

22. Fisher, R. B., *Lord Lister, 1827–1912* (London, 1977): 194.

23. Howie, W. B. and Black, S. A. B.,, 'Sidelights on Lister: a patient's account of Lister's care', *Journal of the History of Medicine* 1977: 239–51.

24. *Ibid.*

25. *Ibid.*

26. *Ibid.*

27. *Ibid.*

28. *Ibid.*

29. *Ibid.*

30. Fisher, *Lord Lister*: 207–8.

31. Leeson, *Lister as I Knew Him*: 169.

32. Lister, J., *BMJ*, 1875, 2: 769–72.

33. Editorial, *Lancet* 1875, 1: 868.

34. *Ibid.*

35. Cameron, *Joseph Lister: the Friend of Man*: 12.

36. Godlee, *Lord Lister*: 394.

37. Editorial, *BMJ*, 1877, 1: 212.

38. Editorial, *BMJ*, 1877, 1: 277.

39. *Ibid.*

40. Fisher, *Lord Lister*: 237.

41. Shepherd, J., *BMJ*, 1967, 1: 42–4.

42. Godlee, *Lord Lister*: 400–5.

43. *Ibid.*

44. Ogston, A., in Ogston, W. H., ed., *Alexander Ogston, KCVO* (Aberdeen, 1943): 92–5.

45. Ogston, ed., *Alexander Ogston*: 63–85.

46. Annual Report, Aberdeen Royal Infirmary, 1869.

47. Ogston, ed., *Alexander Ogston*: 92–5.

48. *Ibid.*

49. *Ibid.*
50. Devine, T. M., *The Scottish Nation, 1700–2000* (London, 1999): 399.
51. Ogston, A., *Edinburgh Medical Journal* 1877, 22: 782–4.
52. *Ibid.*
53. *Ibid.*
54. Ogston, A., *Archiv für Klinische Chirurgie* 1877, 21: 537–46.
55. Pennington, T. H., *Medical History* 1994, 38: 178–88.
56. Ogston, ed., *Alexander Ogston*: 98–101.
57. Koch, R., *Beiträge zur Biologie der Pflanzen* 1877, 2: 399–434.
58. Ogston, ed., *Alexander Ogston*: 98–101.
59. Macdonald, A. and Smith, G., eds. *The Staphylococci* (Aberdeen, 1981): 9–21.
60. Ogston, A., *BMJ*, 1881, 1: 369–75.
61. *Ibid.*
62. *Ibid.*
63. Ogston, A., *Archiv für Klinische Chirurgie* 1880, 25: 588–99.
64. Ogston, A., *BMJ*, 1881, 1: 369–75.
65. Bulloch, W., Obituary, *Lancet* 1929, 1: 309–10.
66. Ogston, ed., *Alexander Ogston*: 113–40.
67. Ogston, A., *Journal of Anatamy and Physiology* 1882;, 16: 526–67.
68. Bowman, A. K., *Sir William Macewen* (London, 1942): 3.
69. Macewen, W., *Transactions of the Royal Institution* 1912, 20: 546–64.
70. Obituary, Sir William Macewen, *Lancet* 1924, 1: 727–8.
71. *Ibid.*
72. James, C. D. T., *Anaesthesia* 1974, 29: 743–53.
73. Macewen, W., *Glasgow Medical Journal* 1874, 6: 87–99.
74. Lister, J., *Lancet* 1869, 1: 451–5.
75. Comrie, J. B., *History of Scottish Medicine* (London, 1932): 642.
76. Macewen, W., *Glasgow Medical Journal* 1874, 6: 87–99.
77. *Ibid.*
78. Lister, J., Letter to William Macewen, 2 October 1873. In Macewen Archive, Royal College of Physicians and Surgeons of Glasgow.
79. Comrie, *History of Scottish Medicine*: 642.
80. Macewen, W., *Glasgow Medical Journal* 1874, 6: 87–99.
81. Macewen, W., Letter to Dr James Allan, 6 October 1873. In Macewen Archive, Royal College of Physicians and Surgeons of Glasgow.
82. Cameron, *Joseph Lister: the Friend of Man*: 12.
83. Macewen, W., *Osteotomy* (London, 1880): 4.
84. Volkmann, R., *Edinburgh Medical Journal* 1875, 19: 794–9.
85. Macewen, *Osteotomy*: 4.
86. Bowman, *Sir William Macewen*: 63–5.
87. Macewen, W., *Lancet* 1880, 2: 450–2.
88. Macewen, W., *Lancet* 1884, 2: 536–9.
89. Macewen, W., *Lancet* 1880, 2: 450–2.
90. Macewen, W., *Lancet* 1884, 2: 536–9.
91. Bowman, *Sir William Macewen*: 185.

92. Leading article, *Lancet* 1884, 2: 650.
93. Bowman, *Sir William Macewen*: 74.

Chapter 6: A Decade of Movement in Antiseptic and Aseptic Surgery, 1880–1890

1. Morgan, K. O., *Oxford Illustrated History of Britain* (Oxford, 1986): 462, 468.
2. Morgan, D., *The Villages of Aberdeen: Footdee* (Aberdeen, 1993): 170–1.
3. Keith, A., *1000 Years of Aberdeen* (Aberdeen, 1972): 312.
4. Longford, E., *Victoria RI* (London, 1966): 225, 372.
5. Ackroyd, P., *London: the Biography* (London, 2000): 343.
6. Smout, T. C., *Century of the Scottish People* (London, 1987): 42–5, 95–6.
7. Robertson, E., *Glasgow's Doctor: Dr J. B. Russell* (East Linton, 1998): 59.
8. Longford, *Victoria RI*: 225, 372.
9. *Ibid.*
10. Smout, *Century of the Scottish People*: 42–5, 95–6.
11. *Ibid.*
12. Morgan, *Oxford Illustrated History of Britain*: 462, 468.
13. Cartwright, F. F., *Social History of Medicine* (London, 1977): 156.
14. Mahon, B., *The Man who Changed Everything* (Chichester, 2004): 1.
15. 'Darwin', *Encyclopedia Brittanica* 15th edn (Chicago, 1985), vol. 16: 1029.
16. Leeson, J. R., *Lister as I Knew Him* (London, 1927): 23–4.
17. Godlee, R. J., *Lord Lister* (London, 1917): 273–8.
18. Lister, J., *Collected Papers* (Oxford, 1909), vol. I, 335–52.
19. Fisher, R. B., *Joseph Lister, 1827–1912* (London, 1977): 234–9.
20. *Ibid.*
21. *Ibid.*
22. Godlee, *Lord Lister*: 410.
23. Shepherd, J., *BMJ* 1967, 1: 42–4.
24. Godlee, *Lord Lister*: 420.
25. Shepherd, J., *BMJ* 1967, 1: 42–4.
26. Shepherd, J., 'Lister and abdominal surgery', in Poynter, F. H. L., ed., *Medicine and Science in the 1860s* (London, 1965): 110–20.
27. Lister, J., *Lancet* 1878, 1: 5–9.
28. Editorial, *BMJ* 1879, 2: 453.
29. Godlee, *Lord Lister*: 459–60.
30. Godlee, *Lord Lister*: 300–4.
31. Godlee, *Lord Lister*: 326.
32. Royal College of Surgeons of England, *Lives of the Fellows* 1953: 464, 510.
33. Jones, P. F., *Journal of Medical Biography* 2001, 9: 143–50.
34. *Ibid.*
35. Macewen, W., *Lancet* 1884, 2: 536–9.
36. Bowman, A. K., *Sir William Macewen* (London, 1942): 66.
37. von Bruns, V., *Berliner Klinischer Wochenschrift* 1880, 43: 609–11.

38. Jones, P. F., *Journal of Medical Biography* 1995, 3: 201–6.
39. *Ibid.*
40. Schimmelbusch, C., *The Aseptic Treatment of Wounds*, trans. Rake, A. T. (London, 1894).
41. Pennington, T. H., *Medical History* 1995, 39: 35–60.
42. Neuber, G., *Centralblatt fur Chirurgie* 1892, 19: 391–401.
43. Schimmelbusch, *The Aseptic Treatment of Wounds*.
44. Wrench, G. T., *Lord Lister* (London, 1913): 331.
45. Tillmans, H., in Fisher, R. B., *Joseph Lister, 1827–1912* (London, 1977): 300.
46. Obituary, Sir David Ferrier, *Royal Society Proceedings B* 1928, 103, VIII–XVI.
47. Macewen, W., *BMJ* 1888, 2: 302–9.
48. Macewen, W., *Lancet* 1881, 2: 541–3, 581–3.
49. *Ibid.*
50. *Ibid.*
51. *Ibid.*
52. *Ibid.*
53. *Ibid.*
54. Jefferson, G., *Sir William Macewen's Contribution to Neurosurgery* (Glasgow, 1950).
55. Macewen, W., *Lancet* 1881, 2: 541–3, 581–3.
56. *Ibid.*
57. Macewen, W., *BMJ* 1888, 2: 302–9.
58. Jefferson, *Sir William Macewen's Contribution to Neurosurgery.*
59. Editorial, *BMJ* 1888, 2: 322–4.
60. Barr, T., *BMJ* 1888, 2: 472–4.
61. Macewen, W., *Pyogenic Disease of the Brain and Spinal Cord* (Glasgow, 1893).
62. Jefferson, *Sir William Macewen's Contribution to Neurosurgery.*

Chapter 7: Consequences of a Revolution, 1890–1900

1. Lister, J., *Collected Papers* (Oxford, 1909), vol. II: 349–64.
2. Pringle, H., *Australia and New Zealand Journal of Surgery* 1995, 65: 887–9.
3. Wangensteen, O. H. and Wangensteen, S. D., *The Rise of Surgery* (Folkestone, 1978): 148–9.
4. Klebs, A. C., 'Theodor Kocher', *US Naval Medical Bulletin* 1918, 12: 59–63.
5. Moynihan, B., *BMJ* 1917, 2: 168.
6. Bloodgood, J. C., *American Journal of Surgery* 1931, 14: 89–148.
7. *Ibid.*
8. Clapesattle, H., *The Doctors Mayo* (Minneapolis, 1941).
9. Ross, J. A., *The Edinburgh School of Surgery after Lister* (Edinburgh, 1978): 22–31.

10. Robarts, F. H. *Journal of the Royal College of Surgeons of Edinburgh* 1969, 14: 299–315.
11. Ross, *The Edinburgh School of Surgery after Lister*: 162.
12. Stiles, H. J., *Surgery, Gynecology and Obstetrics* 1911, 13: 127–40.
13. *Ibid.*
14. Ross, *The Edinburgh School of Surgery after Lister*: 22–31.
15. McKay, W. J. S., *Lawson Tait* (London, 1922): 15.
16. Tait, L., *BMJ* 1886, 1: 921–3.
17. Shepherd, J. A., *Lancet* 1956, 2: 1301–2.
18. Tait, L., *BMJ* 1883, 1: 300–4.
19. McKay, *Lawson Tait*: 105–18.
20. *Ibid.*: 215–16.
21. *Ibid.*
22. Tait, L., *Lectures on Ectopic Pregnancy* (Birmingham, 1888).
23. *Ibid.*
24. Smith, D. C., *New York State Journal of Medicine* 1986, 86: 571–83.
25. Fitz, R. H., *American Journal of Medical Science* 1886, 92: 321–46.
26. McBurney, C., *New York Medical Journal* 1889, 50: 676–84.
27. Moynihan, B. G. A., *Lancet* 1896, 2: 1806–8.
28. *Ibid.*
29. Riddell, J. S., *Scottish Medical Journal* 1900, 6: 214–22, 238–41.
30. Trombley, S., *Sir Frederick Treves* (London, 1979).
31. *Ibid.*
32. Pledger, G. and Stringer, M. D., *BMJ* 2001, 323: 430–1.
33. Kriege, H., *Berliner Klinischer Wochenschrift* 1892, 29: 1244.
34. Morse, T. H., *Lancet* 1894, 1: 671–3.
35. Moynihan, B. G. A., *Lancet* 1901, 2: 1656–63.
36. Clark, H., *Lancet* 1883, 2: 678–80.
37. *Ibid.*
38. Treves, F., *Intestinal Obstruction*, 2nd edn (London, 1899).
39. Annual Reports, Aberdeen Royal Infirmary, 1882–1907.
40. Levack, I. D. and Dudley, H. A. F., *Aberdeen Royal Infirmary* (London, 1992): 31–44.
41. Pennington, T. H., *Medical History* 1995, 39: 35–60.
42. Annual Reports, Aberdeen Royal Infirmary, 1882–1907.
43. *Ibid.*
44. Levack and Dudley, *Aberdeen Royal Infirmary*: 31–44.
45. Ogston, A., *Reminiscences of Three Campaigns* (London, 1920).
46. *Ibid.*
47. Bowman, A. K., *Sir William Macewen* (London, 1942): 298–345.
48. *Ibid.*
49. *Ibid.*
50. Duguid, C., *Macewen of Glasgow* (Edinburgh, 1957).
51. Fisher, R. B., *Joseph Lister, 1827–1912* (London, 1977), 294–303.
52. Maylard, A. E., 'Lister', in *Lister and the Lister Ward* (Glasgow, 1927): 3–20.

53. Lister, J., Letter to Hector Cameron, 12 April 1893. In Lister Archive, Royal College of Surgeons of Edinburgh.
54. Cameron, H. Charles, *Joseph Lister, the friend of man* (London, 1948): 147–8.
55. Godlee, R. J., *Lord Lister* (London, 1917): 530–1.
56. Lister, J., *BMJ* 1896, 2: 733–41.
57. 'Experiments with Roentgen's rays', *Aberdeen Journal*, 15 February 1896.
58. Annual Reports, Aberdeen Royal Infirmary, 1882–1907.
59. Reid, R., *Marie Curie* (London, 1978).
60. Cameron, H. Clare, *Reminiscences of Lister, 1860–1869* (Glasgow, 1927).
61. Robertson, E., *The Yorkhill Story* (Glasgow, 1972).
62. Maylard, 'Lister': 3–20.
63. Turner, G. G., Obituary, *BMJ* 1929, 1: 50.
64. Cameron, *Reminiscences of Lister*.
65. *Ibid.*
66. Rutherfurd, H., Obituary, *Lancet* 1928, 2: 1162.

Suggestions for Further Reading

A number of memoirs of Joseph Lister were written by those who had known and worked with him. The major biography was assembled by Lister's nephew, Rickman Godlee, during the five years following Lister's death (*Lord Lister*, London, 1917), by which time Godlee was himself a consultant surgeon in London. Although 670 pages long, it is a warm and very readable book. Godlee had spent time with Lister as a student, and then he was his personal assistant for some years. The narrative gains much more from this insight into his subject than any loss there might be from bias. By quoting freely from Lister family papers, Godlee illustrates the strong relationship between Joseph and his father, and they help us to appreciate both the modesty and gentle spirit of the man, which contrasts with the steely determination of his pursuit of the truth.

A slender companion to this book was written by Hector Cameron when he was over 80 – (*Reminiscences of Lister*. Glasgow, 1927). In only 45 pages, he provides a memorable picture of his hero, with some good anecdotes. Cameron was Lister's house surgeon during 1867, and then his personal assistant through the years in Glasgow when the antiseptic system was born.

J. R. Leeson in *Lister as I Knew Him* (London, 1927) wrote from the unusual position of a London medical student who elected to visit Lister while he was Professor in Edinburgh. Leeson recalls the details of his visit to Lister at his home, to present his credentials, and records vivid memories of the smells, sights and sounds of the crowded wards and operating amphitheatre of the Surgical Hospital.

Hector Cameron's son, Charles, had become a paediatrician at Guy's Hospital, London, when he wrote *Joseph Lister: the Friend of Man* (London, 1948). He recalls childhood memories of Lister's visits to his father in Glasgow. Then as a medical student in London he would call on the Listers in their London home, and share in Lister's reminiscences. Charles provides an affectionate account of the lifelong friendship which grew up between Lister and Cameron.

R. B. Fisher, in a modern biography, *Joseph Lister, 1827–1912* (London, 1977), draws on his extensive researches in the records of the Lister family, which were not available to earlier writers. Its 330 pages provide an important contribution to the Lister literature.

The main source of material on Alexander Ogston is the memoir assembled by his family – *Sir Alexander Ogston, KCVO*, edited by his son Walter, and published privately. It contains many tributes by family and friends and, most importantly, 'Scattered Recollections'. These are autobiographical notes which give vivid snapshots of his life as a student in Scotland and Europe, as a young graduate, and in later professional life. Ogston's three bacteriological papers are remarkably detailed, and give a unique insight into the improvisations which led to his discoveries, which were made during the birth of the science of bacteriology. The centenary of this work was celebrated in a conference, which was reported in *The Staphylococci* (ed. A Macdonald and G. Smith, Aberdeen, 1981). This contains full reviews of Ogston's life, especially his activities during retirement.

In his preface to *Sir William Macewen* (London, 1942), A.K. Bowman quotes his subject in saying 'a surgeon must be a physician. Otherwise he is little more than an amateur mechanic.' Bowman hoped that this would justify him, a physician, in tackling a surgical biography. Allowing for some favouritism – as an old student – Bowman gives a full and fair account of an extraordinary career. He was fortunate to have the assistance of Macewen's daughter, Margaret, who provided some excellent anecdotes. The Macewen Memorial Lectures offer some thoughtful contributions, particularly those of Professors Grey Turner (1939) and Geoffrey Jefferson (1950).

The Edinburgh School of Surgery after Lister (Edinburgh, 1978), by James A. Ross, is a valuable source of information on surgeons and surgical practice for the fifty years after 1877.

Index